P9-BYG-582

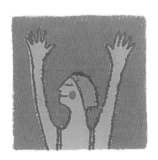

SHAPING UP

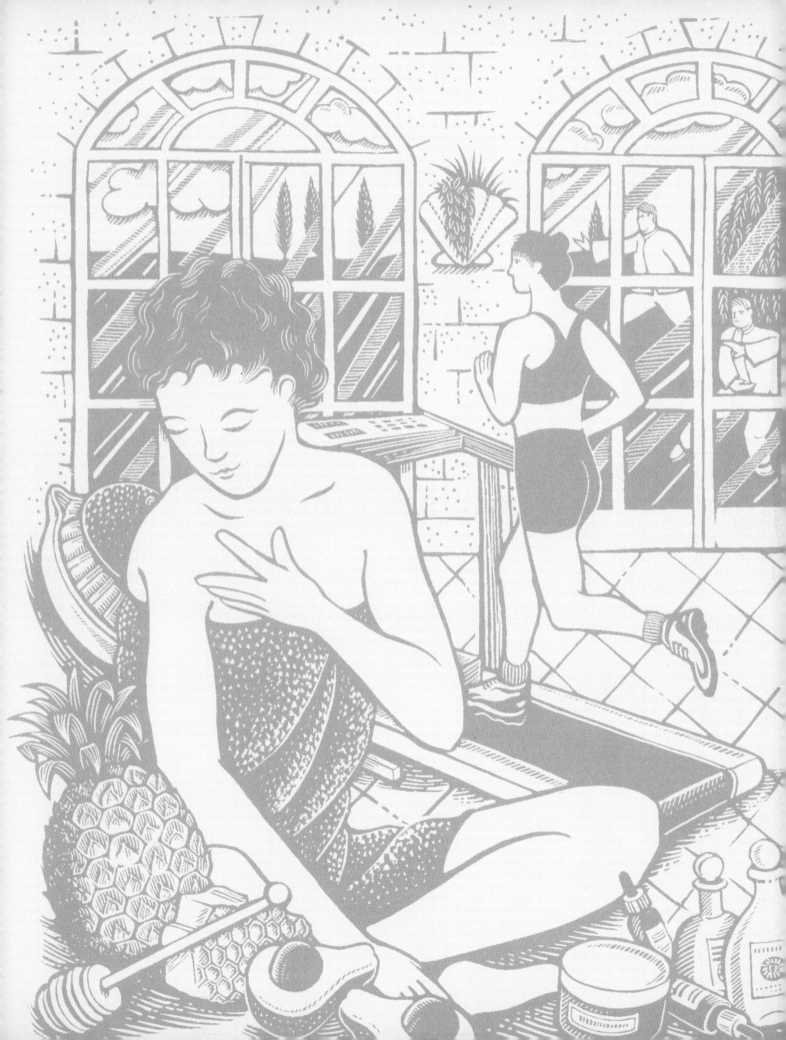

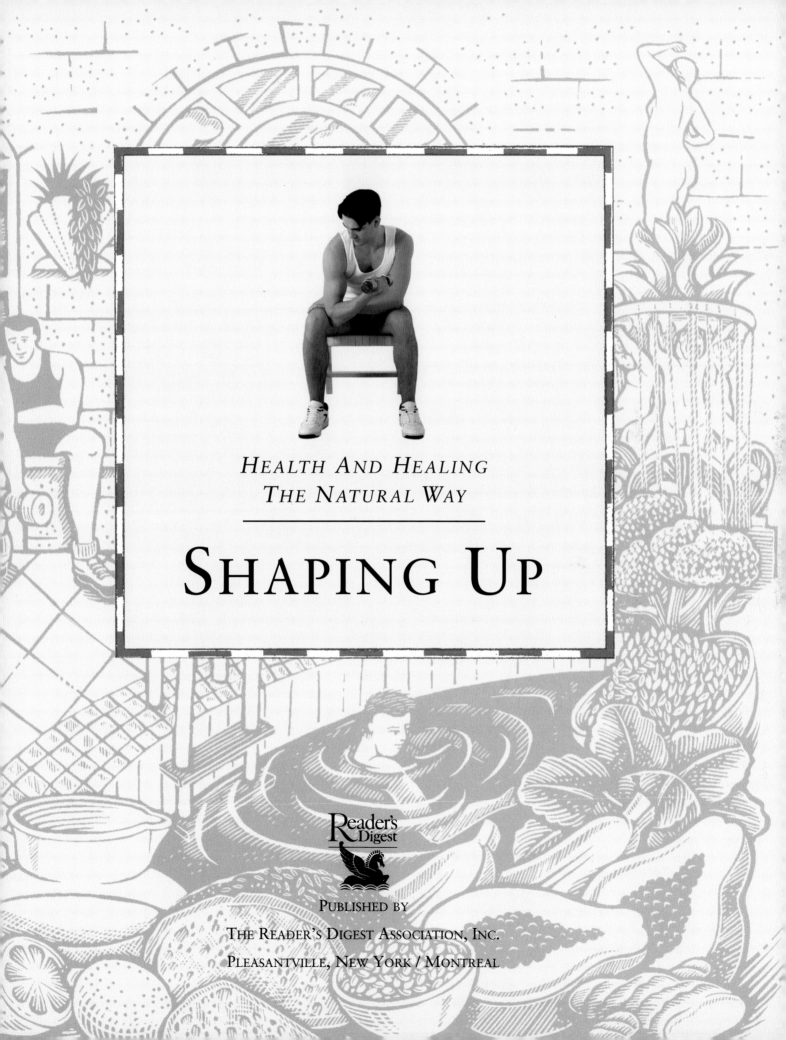

HEALTH AND HEALING
THE NATURAL WAY

SHAPING UP

Reader's
Digest

PUBLISHED BY

THE READER'S DIGEST ASSOCIATION, INC.

PLEASANTVILLE, NEW YORK / MONTREAL

A READER'S DIGEST BOOK
produced by
Carroll & Brown Limited, London

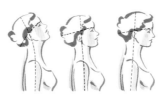

CARROLL & BROWN

Publishing Director Denis Kennedy
Art Director Chrissie Lloyd

Managing Editor Sandra Rigby
Managing Art Editor Tracy Timson

Editors Joanne Stanford, Richard Emerson,
Caroline Uzielli

Designers Sandra Brooke,
Vimit Punater, Julie Bennett

Photographers Jules Selmes, David Murray

Production Wendy Rogers, Karen Kloot

Computer Management John Clifford, Paul Stradling,
Elisa Merino

Copyright © 2000 The Reader's Digest Association, Inc.
Copyright © 2000 The Reader's Digest Association (Canada) Ltd.
Copyright © 2000 Reader's Digest Association Far East Ltd.
Philippine Copyright © 2000 Reader's Digest Association Far East Ltd.

All rights reserved. Unauthorized reproduction,
in any manner, is prohibited.

® Reader's Digest and the Pegasus logo are
registered trademarks of The Reader's Digest Association, Inc.

Printed in the United States of America

Library of Congress Cataloging in Publication Data

Shaping Up
        p. cm. — (Health and healing the natural way)
    Includes index
    ISBN 0-7621-0282-9
      1. Exercise 2. Physical fitness
    I. Reader's Digest Association. II. Series.

RA781 .S525 2000
613.7—dc21
                                        00-020388

CONSULTANTS

Malcolm Whyatt D.Phy., M.A.I.C.
Publisher and Editor, Health and Strength Magazine,
Hereford, England
Mike Fish MSc and John Orum BSc
Optimus Fitness Consultancy

MEDICAL ILLUSTRATIONS CONSULTANT

Amanda Roberts MA, MB, BChir

CONTRIBUTORS

Jane Griffin BSc (Nutrition), SRD
Nutritional and Dietetic Consultant
Professor Rozalind Gruben AHSI, RSA
Health and Fitness Consultant
Claire Hill
Medical Health Writer
Anita Kleijn BA Hons
Natural Health and Fitness Consultant

READER'S DIGEST PROJECT STAFF

Series Editor Gayla Visalli
Editorial Director, Health & Medicine Wayne Kalyn
Associate Designer Jennifer R. Tokarski
Production Technology Manager Douglas A. Croll
Editorial Manager Christine R. Guido

READER'S DIGEST ILLUSTRATED REFERENCE BOOKS

Editor-in-Chief Christopher Cavanaugh
Art Director Joan Mazzeo
Operations Manager William J. Cassidy

Address any comments about *Shaping Up* to
Editor-in-Chief, U.S. Illustrated Reference Books,
Pleasantville, NY 10570

The information in this book is for reference only;
it is not intended as a substitute for a doctor's diagnosis and care.
The editors urge anyone with continuing medical problems
or symptoms to consult a doctor.

SHAPING UP

More and more people today are choosing to take greater responsibility for their own health care rather than relying on a doctor to step in with a cure when something goes wrong. We now recognize that we can influence our health by making improvements in lifestyle, for example, eating better, getting more exercise, and reducing stress. People are also becoming increasingly aware that there are other healing methods—some of them new, others ancient—that can help prevent illness or be used as a complement to orthodox medicine.

The series *Health and Healing the Natural Way* can help you to make your own health choices by giving you clear, comprehensive, straightforward, and encouraging information and advice about methods of improving your health. The series explains the many different natural therapies that are now available, including aromatherapy, herbalism, acupressure, and a number of others, and the circumstances in which they may be of benefit when used in conjunction with conventional medicine.

Feeling at ease with yourself and your appearance can have a great influence on your health and well-being, giving you the confidence to live life to the fullest. *SHAPING UP* aims to help you make the most of your body by showing you how to boost your fitness and improve your physical appearance at the same time. Because a well-balanced diet is important to maintaining a good shape, the book examines the rules of healthy eating. And because exercise for muscular strength and flexibility offers a sure path to a fitter, firmer body, *SHAPING UP* provides comprehensive instructions and step-by-step illustrations for a range of exercise techniques and routines. The book also looks at how some alternative therapies view body shape and gives you insight into what shape and posture can tell you about yourself and others. It provides suggestions as well for alternative exercises, from t'ai chi to salsa, to help you achieve your full potential.

CONTENTS

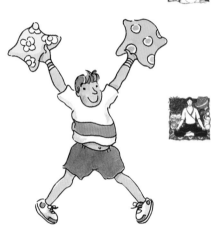

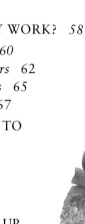

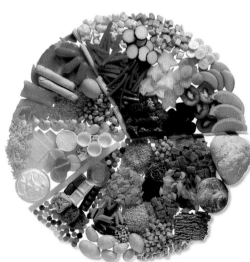

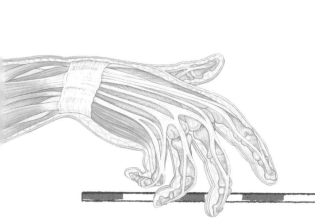

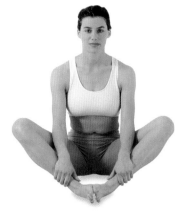

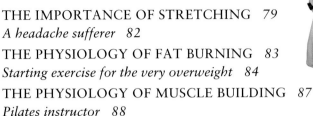

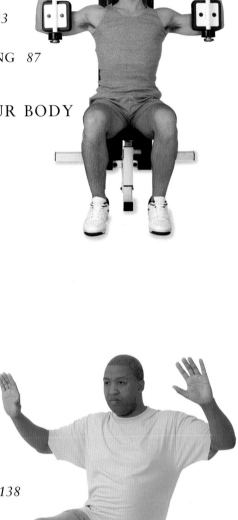

 5 EXERCISES TO SHAPE UP YOUR BODY

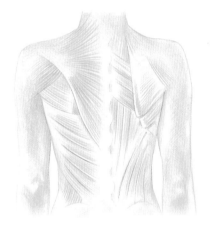

 6 ALTERNATIVE WAYS OF SHAPING UP

A HEALTHY SHAPE

The most effective way to achieve your best possible body shape is to combine a well-balanced diet with the right kind of exercise and a good mental attitude.

Western society has always placed importance on the appearance of the human body. From ancient art to contemporary images in magazines, art, and other media, the depiction of an ideally shaped human body has been an almost constant theme and one that has enormous psychological effects upon us as observers.

In practice, artists distort reality to reflect the prevailing concept of beauty in their own culture and society. The fact that an artist's concept of perfection has often been extremely difficult or even impossible for real men and women to achieve is irrelevant. For example, the ancient Greek sculptor Zeuxis reputedly carved a statue of Venus using five women as models and taking the most beautiful aspect from each to create an ideal whole. In the same way, in order to create their perfect picture, contemporary advertisers manipulate images by improving tans, smoothing away blemishes and bumps, and using flattering angles. The purpose is not to create high art but an appealing image, one that will make us want to buy the product being promoted.

In recent years society's prevailing concept of perfect shape has been questioned. Increasingly, common disorders like anorexia and bulimia have made us aware of how the desire for an ideal body shape can become a dangerous obsession. The notion of an attractive body has now come to include a much broader concept of overall good health, fitness, and general well-being.

THE SEARCH FOR A PERFECT SHAPE

The ancient Greeks were the first people to develop fully and systematically the concept of the perfect human form, and Greek ideals still continue to influence us today. Between 480 and 440 B.C. Greek artists perfected the representation of the human form, but they did not base their art purely on detailed observation of nature. Rather, Greek statues embodied the principles of mathematical proportion that were so important to the Greek culture in general. The Greeks had great faith in harmonious numbers, which they

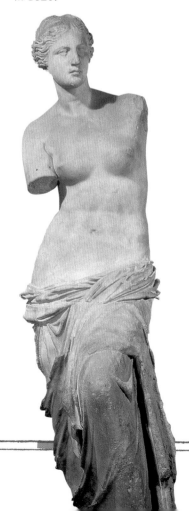

VENUS DE MILO
This marble statue from ancient Greece, dating from around 100 B.C., has been a world-renowned symbol of beauty since her discovery in 1820.

believed governed nature, including the shape of the human body. The perfect human shape should conform to a series of measurable proportions, which could be mathematically calculated. Some of these rules of proportion have survived and been passed down to us. For example, art scholars can observe in Greek sculpture that the head is the basis of proportion for the rest of the body, with a man being seven and a half heads high and a woman seven heads high. The measurement between a woman's breasts is one head length, from breast to navel also a head length, and this distance is equal to that from the navel to the crotch.

Another clue to Greek rules of human proportion is found in the writings of the Roman scholar Vitruvius. One of his most famous statements was that a temple should have the proportions of a man. He added that a man's body is a model of proportion because with arms and legs extended it fits into the perfect geometrical forms of the square and circle. This statement obsessed Renaissance artists, but following Vitruvius's dictates to the letter resulted in images of the body that look very odd: the feet, arms, and legs are overly long and the resulting figure has more in common with the proportions of a gorilla than those of a man or a woman. This was one of the first, although certainly not the last, examples of how difficult or even impossible it is for people to measure up to ideals of proportion.

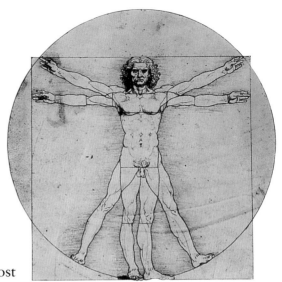

PERFECT PROPORTIONS?
Vitruvius's statement that the ideal body corresponds to geometrical shapes fascinated Renaissance artists. This drawing by Leonardo da Vinci was one of the more successful attempts to illustrate the dictum.

ATHLETIC ABILITIES
Like the Greeks before us, we strive to take our bodies to the limit of their athletic capabilities with competitions like the Olympic games.

THE UNION OF MIND, BODY, AND SPIRIT

Although shape was important to the Greeks, physical beauty meant far more than simply creating an object that pleased the eye. An ideal form represented a harmonious union of the finest aspects of the body, mind, and spirit. A beautiful body represented physical strength and prowess, important characteristics in a society affected by war and physical danger. Athletes and athletic games held a high status in Greek society, and outstanding performers were honored for their achievements.

In perfect form the Greeks also celebrated the beauty of reason because harmonious mathematical proportions represented by the finest physical specimens displayed the triumph of the intellect and logic. A beautiful body revealed the fundamental principles upon which Greek scholars believed the world rested.

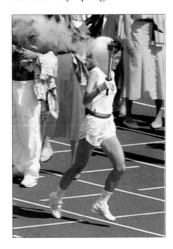

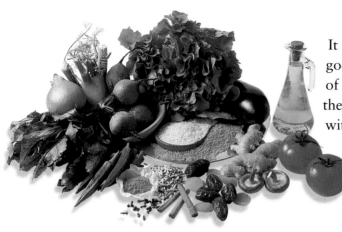

It is also significant that the Greeks chose to depict their gods, the representatives of spiritual concerns, in the form of idealized humans. Both male and female sculptures of the 5th century B.C. depicted gods as physically powerful, with rippling muscles, broad shoulders, and powerful necks. They emerge as athletes and warriors, competitors in Pan-Hellenic games. To the Greeks, perfect shape united and symbolized the harmonious interaction of mind, body, and spirit.

THE KAPHA DIET
According to Ayurvedic principles, your diet should be customized to balance or calm your dominant dosha. The foods shown here are recommended for kapha types, who put on weight easily and should avoid too many sweet or fatty foods.

NATURAL ALIGNMENT
Young children naturally hold their spines erect. Unfortunately, as we age we tend to lose this innate sense of body alignment. Body-reading therapies propose to help you regain your natural posture.

SHAPE AND WHO WE ARE

The concept of a pleasing shape signifying more than aesthetic beauty is not an exclusively Greek idea. It is reflected in many cultures and belief systems, including traditional Chinese medicine, Ayurvedic medicine, and other healing systems used by people around the world.

Ayurveda, the ancient medical practice of India, means "life knowledge," and this knowledge comes primarily from observing body shape. Ayurvedic medicine assumes a very close alliance among body type and personality, spirituality, and the potential for health or disease. The system divides people into three general body types. A *vata* person is generally slim, quick moving, energetic, and perhaps prone to anxiety or nervous disorders. A *pitta* type has a medium build and coloring and is quick to anger if provoked. *Kapha* describes a large-framed person, who is likely to be slow to show emotions or worry. From observing a person's shape and determining his or her dominant type, an Ayurvedic practitioner can identify behavior or symptoms that clash with the natural type, such as a normally energetic vata type being overcome with fatigue and lethargy, and thus diagnose related health problems. The body shapes are seen as manifestations of basic energy forces that are present throughout the world, and in different combinations they define the personalities of individuals.

The idea that the physical body is linked with mental and spiritual health is also central to some modern healing systems, such as Rolfing and the Alexander technique, both devised in the 20th century. These therapies incorporate the idea that your body stance reflects deeply held emotional stresses and traumas. Therapists argue that such signs as a tense or hunched posture, imbalance in the proportions of the upper and lower body, or persistent muscular pain point to deeper problems, and that improving body shape through changes in posture or massage and manipulation will help to address these issues. In Rolfing and Hellerwork the muscles and bones are massaged and manipulated to release tension and promote well-being. The Alexander technique concentrates on posture and how to use your body with minimum effort and maximum efficiency. Many people find they gain increased self-awareness and self-confidence while undergoing physical therapy with these techniques.

DIET AND SHAPE

A healthy diet is a vital part of a shaping-up program; it is essential to understand how to fuel your body correctly. Many people who want to lose weight think that reducing their food intake is the answer. Starving yourself is not the way to long-term weight control. While portions are important, the types of food eaten, not just the quantity, are also key elements. A healthy mix of fruits and vegetables, whole grains, and lean protein and a limited intake of fatty and sugary foods will keep your body and immune system strong and help you lose weight gradually. Fruits and vegetables also provide important nutrients for a radiant skin; for example, avocados are rich in essential fatty acids, while strawberries, oranges, and raspberries can enhance your skin's natural regenerative properties. Regular aerobic exercise will also help you to achieve your weight-loss goals, but before starting an exercise regimen, you should understand your body's basic energy requirements to ensure that you maintain your vitality.

WHY SHOULD WE SHAPE UP?

Good shape is not just about looking good; it should also reflect good health—physically, mentally, and spiritually. As both the ancient Greeks and Ayurvedic practitioners discovered, these aspects are inextricably linked: emotional strain takes its toll on the body just as much as physical injuries or pain do. A healthy lifestyle is one that addresses diet, exercise, and issues of emotional health in recognition that there is no split between your mind and body.

Regular physical exercise will help to control your weight, improving the ratio of muscle to fat and increasing your metabolic rate so that you burn calories faster. At the same time it will

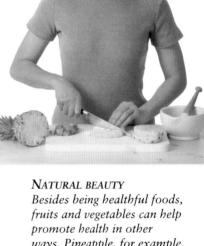

NATURAL BEAUTY
Besides being healthful foods, fruits and vegetables can help promote health in other ways. Pineapple, for example, can be cut into small pieces, mashed using a pestle and mortar, and mixed with yogurt to create a face pack that improves problem skin.

TONING THE BODY
Inches can be lost just by toning up the muscles of your body. This is particularly true of the stomach, which can be tightened with specific exercises such as this oblique curl (see page 127).

bring about major benefits for your general health, including enhancement of the efficiency of your cardiovascular system and improvement in your strength and mobility. Exercise will also benefit the tone and condition of your skin because it improves circulation. Finally, exercise has a well-documented positive effect on mood, releasing the mood-enhancing chemicals endorphins.

To some extent we are all limited by our genetically inherited shape: we are tall or short, large framed or petite, have a tendency to store fat or be thin, according to our genetic makeup and the environment in which we grew up. However, research has shown that regardless of our bone and muscle structure, we can all make huge improvements in our health and well-being, and ultimately how we look, by addressing certain lifestyle factors.

DANCING INTO SHAPE
Not everyone relishes the idea of going to a gym to work out, but luckily there are many options for toning your body. Dancing is one that can be particularly enjoyable.

SHAPING UP AS PART OF YOUR LIFE

Most people are now aware of the importance of including exercise and a healthy diet in their lifestyle, but they become confused or discouraged if they do not change shape as much as they would like or expect through an exercise program. *SHAPING UP* explains the specific types of exercise that help to define muscle tone and create a more defined outline to the body. Once the underlying principles to shaping up are understood, it is relatively easy to include them in your daily life to achieve a better, stronger body. Chapter 1 looks at the importance of a healthy body and shape and analyzes the basic body types we conform to. It also discusses how the culture in which we were brought up and our diet during our growing years may influence our shape. Chapter 2 looks at Ayurveda and other body-reading therapies that link shape with emotional health. Chapter 3 examines wider lifestyle issues that contribute to the overall physical impression you create, from eating healthfully for a better body shape to taking good care of your skin to choosing the most flattering clothes. Chapter 4 explains in detail the principles of fat burning and muscle toning, and will help you to develop a personalized program to achieve your goals. Chapter 5 provides a comprehensive program of exercises that you can follow to tone, stretch, and strengthen all your muscles. Most of these exercises can be easily performed in the comfort of your own home. Finally, Chapter 6 looks at different ways in which you can shape up using ancient techniques such as yoga and t'ai chi, as well as different forms of dance.

WOULD YOU BENEFIT FROM A SHAPING-UP PROGRAM?

Even if you are not overweight and do not feel the need to change your diet, you may still be unfit in other ways and therefore can benefit from shaping up. It has been shown that older adults who are physically active have the stamina of sedentary people who are 10 to 20 years younger. By undertaking a program to increase your strength and muscular fitness, you will see benefits that go far beyond uncovering a firmer, more defined body.

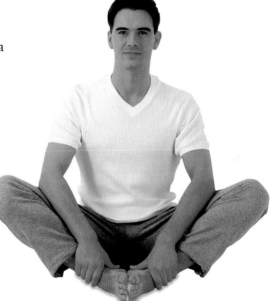

Q **DO YOU WISH YOU LOOKED MORE LIKE MODELS IN MAGAZINES?**

They may look stunning, but many of the images that we see in magazines have been electronically altered to disguise imperfections and sometimes to make arms and legs appear longer and thinner. It is important to recognize that the images of popular culture are not necessarily practical or even possible to emulate. Cultural perceptions are often very difficult to challenge, but improving your shape and strength by doing the right exercises should make you feel more confident about your body. (See Chapter 1.)

Q **DO YOUR MUSCLES AND BONES ACHE IF YOU ARE STRESSED OR TENSE?**

Our body language is extremely important. Often emotional stresses that we do not consciously admit to in our everyday lives show up in our bodies. Hunched shoulders, a clenched jaw, or tightly crossed legs could mask feelings of frustration, insecurity, or chronic stress. Body therapy to unknot muscles or correct bad posture that has built up over a period of time, sometimes even years, can help to release and overcome past stresses or emotional trauma. (See Chapter 2.)

Q **DO YOU EXERCISE REGULARLY BUT STILL THINK YOU LOOK TOO BULKY?**

Although it is essential to exercise to improve the efficiency of your cardiovascular system, many of the muscles you build up by running or playing a game like squash may give you bulky muscles and not improve your suppleness. It is important to include some sort of stretching in your exercise program to encourage muscles to lengthen and to increase your flexibility. (See Chapter 4.)

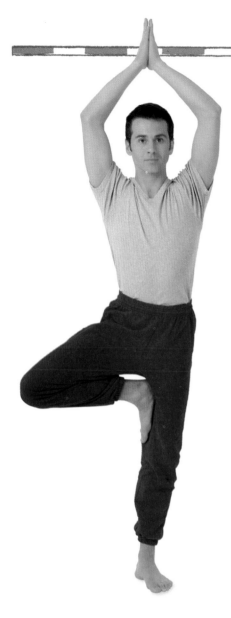

Q DO YOU FIND IT DIFFICULT TO MAKE TIME FOR EXERCISE IN YOUR LIFE?

Many people find it very difficult to make time for regular exercise. Juggling the demands of children, work, and partners can be all-consuming, and exercise frequently ends up being neglected. However, many toning and strengthening exercises can be performed while seated at your desk working or even while watching television. Exercise can become part of your social life as well; for example, dancing classes will give you opportunities for socializing in addition to toning and shaping. Exercise can also contribute to relaxation and stress relief. Many people are unaware of the extent to which yoga, for instance, can build muscle tone while providing relief from stress. Chapter 5 includes exercises that can be performed at home or at work, and Chapter 6 provides easy-to-follow alternative regimens for shaping up.

Q DO YOU WANT TO SHAPE UP BUT HATE THE IDEA OF WEIGHT TRAINING AND OTHER SPORTS?

Participating in a sport and doing regular resistance exercise with weights are very effective ways to shape up, but they are not the only possibilities available. There are many alternative methods that you can use to improve the flexibility and strength of your muscles and bones, from ancient regimens such as yoga and t'ai chi, to dance classes or even just walking back from the store with shopping bags on a regular basis instead of using the car or taking a bus. When you understand the principles of shaping up you can include a variety of activities in your life that will contribute to your goal. (See Chapter 6.)

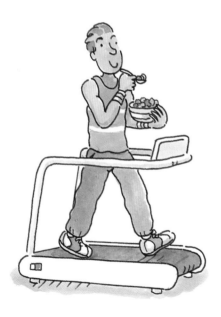

Q ARE YOU CONSTANTLY TRYING NEW DIETS BUT DO NOT SEEM TO BE ABLE TO CHANGE YOUR SHAPE?

Eating healthy low-fat food is only a small part of shaping up. Dieting will eventually reduce the amount of fat in your body but it will not tone your muscles. If you do not exercise at the same time, your body may remain flabby, especially if you lose a great deal of weight. In order to tone your body, you need to develop some sort of exercise program while introducing dietary change. However, change doesn't necessarily mean a reduction in the amount of food you eat: reducing high-fat and sugary foods and including more whole grains, low-fat protein, and fruits and vegetables will help to control your weight while ensuring you don't go hungry. Chapter 3 provides advice on healthy eating, while Chapter 4 explains the principles of fat burning and muscle toning.

CHAPTER 1

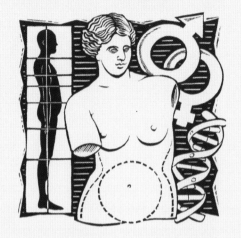

YOUR BODY SHAPE

Many factors affect our shape, including diet, exercise, age, sex, and genetic inheritance; even our emotions can influence the shape of our bodies. Successful shaping up involves recognizing not only what you perhaps can and should try to change about your body but also those aspects of your shape that you must learn to accept.

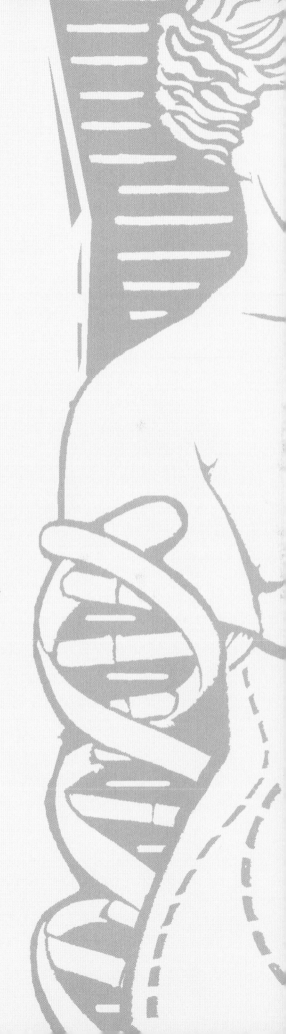

THE IMPORTANCE OF A HEALTHY SHAPE

Society's notion of the ideal body shape can veer dangerously away from one that is healthy, so before beginning to shape up, make sure you know what a healthy shape means for you.

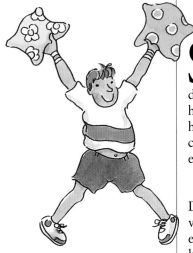

WHY EXERCISE?
Exercise is not just about increasing muscle strength or losing weight. Numerous health benefits, including reduced risk of serious conditions such as heart disease and some forms of cancer should inspire even the most confirmed couch potato.

Society today encourages us to be highly conscious of body shape. Books, magazines, and television shows all advocate diets and exercise programs designed to help us achieve a slim, attractive figure. But how realistic are our expectations for changing our shape, and what do health experts recommend as a healthy goal?

WEIGHT AND SHAPE

Dietitians and doctors see a healthy shape as very much related to a healthy weight. The evidence is clear: serious illnesses, such as heart disease and diabetes, are far more common among the obese. Obesity can also lead to respiratory problems, such as breathlessness and asthma, as well as circulatory and blood problems—anemia and varicose veins,

for example. If you are overweight and also smoke or drink, losing weight can be even more crucial in reducing the likelihood of developing a serious health condition.

You can find out whether you are within the recommended weight range for your height by calculating your Body Mass Index, or BMI (see below). It is a good idea also to have your body fat measured. More than 33 percent fat is unhealthy for women; more than 25 percent fat is unhealthy for men.

If your BMI puts you in the overweight or obese category, consult your doctor about how to combine dietary change and exercise to best achieve your goals and make sure that you don't undertake exercise that could place a sudden strain on your body and perhaps precipitate a heart attack.

CALCULATING YOUR BODY MASS INDEX

Because the Body Mass Index (BMI) is a respected gauge for healthy weight, you should check your BMI before starting a weight-loss plan. You may find that a desirable weight as indicated by your BMI is lower than that mandated in weight and height charts created by insurance companies. Instructions are given below for how to find your BMI.

1 *Weigh yourself in kilograms (to convert pounds into kilograms, divide your weight in pounds by 2.2).*

2 *Measure your height in meters (to convert from inches to meters, multiply your height in inches by 0.025).*

3 *Square your height (multiply your height by your height).*

4 *Divide your weight by your squared height (see example, below).*

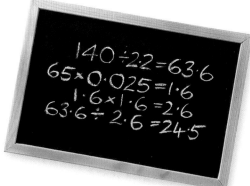

IS YOUR BMI HEALTHY?
A healthy BMI score is between 20 and 25. Under 20 is classed as underweight; over 25 is overweight; and over 30 is considered obese.

HEALTH GAINS FOR EVERYONE

Even if you are the correct weight for your height, you should still exercise regularly for the benefit of your general health. Exercise can improve the functioning of the cardiovascular system, making the heart pump more efficiently, and it can help to lower high blood pressure and improve cholesterol levels in the blood. Research has shown that regular exercise, even after a long period of inactivity, reduces the risk of heart attack and stroke and can help in the management of many diseases, such as arthritis and diabetes.

Regular exercise will also improve your general well-being. It not only is a good stress reducer but also increases your energy level, lifts your mood, and promotes sound sleep. Current guidelines recommend that, regardless of age, you should exercise at least three times a week for at least 20 minutes at a level that raises your heart rate.

BASIC BODY TYPES

Despite the wide variety of shapes and sizes that occur, most people correspond to one of three basic body shapes. Recognizing which category you fall into can help you plan a shaping-up program that takes into account the challenges that your particular body type poses.

In the 1940s W. H. Sheldon of Harvard University was the first person to use the terms *ectomorph, mesomorph,* and *endomorph.* He was primarily interested in linking body shapes and personality types. Today, however, his classifications are used mainly to identify physiological patterns and tendencies. Some fitness experts advise that certain types of exercise are more suitable for particular body types.

Ectomorphs

Ectomorphs are generally tall and thin. Their legs are usually long in proportion to their torso, and they have a strong bone structure. These people find it hard to put on weight when they are young, but tend to fill out a little with age. When they do gain weight, it is usually evenly distributed over the whole body. Following a balanced diet but increasing the intake of starchy carbohydrates will prevent ectomorphs from becoming too thin when they exercise. Types of exercise that particularly suit ectomorphs include ballet, marathon running, cycling, aerobic dance, and weight training.

Endomorphs

Endomorphs are more curvaceous and shorter than ectomorphs and have a tendency to gain body fat easily, which they often store around the abdomen. Their legs tend to be short in proportion to their torso, and they have the heaviest bone structure of the three types. A sensible diet that is low in fat is important for them. Types of exercise that suit endomorphs include cycling, walking, swimming, and low-impact aerobics.

Mesomorphs

Mesomorphs are of medium height and build, as a rule, with a strong and muscular frame. Their legs are about the same length as their torso. Women with this shape tend to have hips larger than their shoulders and gain weight first around their thighs and then their hips and buttocks. Mesomorphs can put on weight easily, but because they also build muscle easily, a moderate amount of regular exercise is usually enough to keep their body shape under control. In terms of exercise, mesomorphs do well with weight training, circuit training, martial arts, skiing, and racket sports.

These three basic body shapes are largely determined by genetic inheritance; your body shape will inevitably take after that of

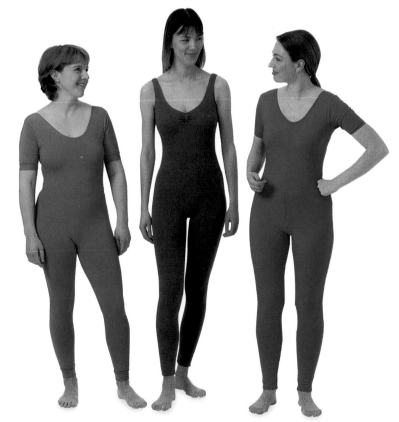

YOUR BODY SHAPE
The three basic body shapes—endomorph (left), ectomorph (middle), and mesomorph (right)—give clues as to how your body distributes weight. This information can help you to plan a diet and exercise program that targets your problem areas.

APPLE AND PEAR SHAPES

Depending on how their bodies store fat, people fall into two main body shapes—apple and pear. Research has shown that apple-shaped people may be more easily disposed to heart disease and cancer, so it is important for them to keep their weight in check with diet and exercise. Menopausal women tend to be apple shaped because of hormonal changes that cause weight gain mainly in the abdominal area.

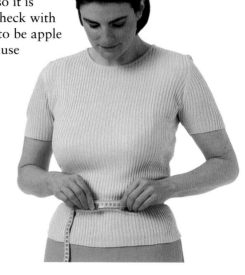

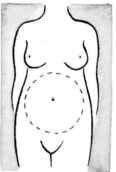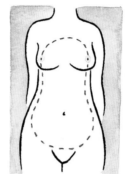

FAT DISTRIBUTION
"Apples" are round in shape and have little waist definition. They tend to store fat around the abdomen. "Pears" tend to store weight around the buttocks and thighs.

ARE YOU APPLE SHAPED?
Divide your waist measurement in inches by your hip measurement in inches. If the answer is more than 0.8, you are an apple shape.

someone in your family (see page 26). There is little you can do to change your basic shape—some of us are tall, and nothing we do will make us smaller. However, there is a lot you can do to better your shape by improving your posture (see Chapter 2) and increasing overall fitness and flexibility (see Chapters 4 and 5). You can also create visual tricks with clothing to appear shorter, taller, or more slender (see pages 71–74).

POSTURE AND ALIGNMENT

Health experts agree that a healthy body shape encompasses not only weight and fat distribution but also good posture and alignment. There are a number of therapies that are concerned with the excess stress incorrect posture and body misalignment can place on muscles and joints. Poor posture can be implicated in back pain, as well as neck and shoulder problems. Therapists

STEPS TOWARD A BETTER BODY SHAPE
If you are unhappy with your body shape, whether or not you are overweight, the psychological effects can result in poor self-image. Deciding that it's time for a change could be the best decision of your life, improving both your health and happiness.

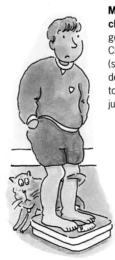

Make an informed choice about your goal before you start. Check your BMI (see page 16) to decide if you need to lose weight or just tone up.

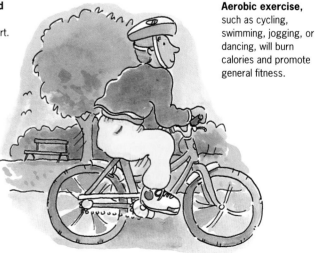

Aerobic exercise, such as cycling, swimming, jogging, or dancing, will burn calories and promote general fitness.

who specialize in manipulating the body into better alignment will analyze how you stand and walk, looking for imbalances and misalignments in your body in order to help determine effective treatment.

Many body-reading therapies, such as the Alexander technique with its system of movement reeducation, focus on posture as the linchpin of good health. Practitioners believe that correct posture not only relieves muscle tension but also improves the functioning of internal organs. In addition, therapies like Rolfing and Hellerwork work to release pent-up emotions (see pages 47–50).

The idea of posture and alignment being linked to emotions has been recognized by traditional Eastern approaches to health for thousands of years. The ancient Indian health system of Ayurveda, for example, uses analysis of body shape as one of its diagnostic tools (see page 42). Practitioners believe that body shape reveals as much about general physical health as psychological states. (Chapter 2 examines body reading and alignment in greater detail.)

ACHIEVING A HEALTHY SHAPE

Following a sensible diet, exercising regularly, and paying close attention to your posture are the best ways to make the most of your natural shape and to maintain it. Although you can do a lot on your own to improve your posture, you may benefit from seeing a professional teacher of the Alexander technique, a physiotherapist, or a Rolfer to correct physical misalignments. However, everyone can introduce exercise into their lives without the aid of an expert. Any form of exercise will help you to burn

calories and improve your fitness, but some types of exercise will target your shaping-up goals better than others.

Aerobic exercise—any activity that raises your heart rate for at least 12 minutes at a time—will improve the efficiency of your heart and lungs. Aerobic exercise tends to burn calories more effectively than other forms of exercise; in the long term it will improve your general level of fitness, which will allow you to exercise longer and with greater stamina. Examples of aerobic exercise are brisk walking, jogging, cycling, dancing, and swimming.

Flexibility exercises, including yoga and dance, will improve your range of movement. Strength exercises tend to focus more on muscle definition and toning. A whole range of floor and weight-training exercises can improve strength and muscle tone. Chapter 5 looks at these in detail. For alternative forms of exercise that will tone and strengthen muscles, see Chapter 6.

Whatever exercise you choose, it helps to be as informed as possible about how your body works and how you can best improve its efficiency (Chapter 4 provides such information). Reducing the amount of fat stored by your body or building stronger, more toned muscles is not simply a question of exercising; a healthy balanced diet is an essential component to any shaping-up program. Reorienting your diet away from high-fat and high-sugar foods and toward complex carbohydrates and lean protein will improve your long-term health and, in the short term, provide your body with the right energy sources to get in shape (see Chapter 3).

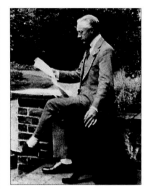

F. M. ALEXANDER (1869–1955)
An Australian actor, F. Matthias Alexander invented his now well-known Alexander technique when he discovered that the voice loss he experienced on stage was linked to a change in his posture brought on by stage fright (see pages 47–48).

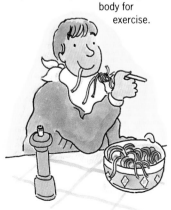

Cutting down on sugary foods and increasing lean protein and complex carbohydrates will fuel your body for exercise.

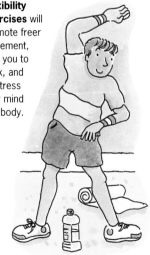

Flexibility exercises will promote freer movement, help you to relax, and de-stress your mind and body.

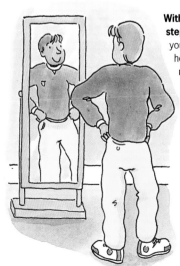

With the positive steps you have taken, you will begin to feel healthier and have more energy and increased self-confidence within a few weeks of starting your program.

The Rolfer

Rolfing is a form of deep-tissue massage that treats the body as a whole with the aim of restructuring and balancing. Within a shaping-up program, it is useful for improving posture and gaining greater flexibility and ease of movement.

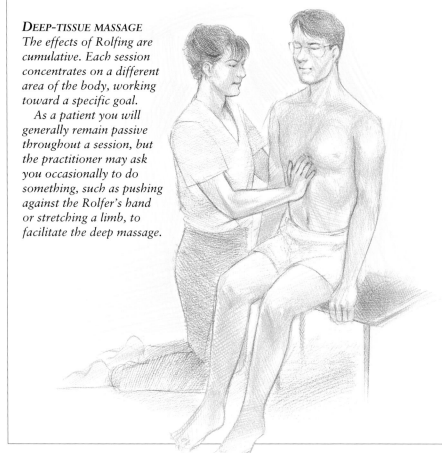

THE ROLF LINE
These pictures form the international Rolfing logo. Rolfers view the body in segments; when all these segments are balanced in relation to each other and within the force of gravity, the body is properly aligned. An imaginary line can then be drawn through the balanced body; this is known as the Rolf Line.

DEEP-TISSUE MASSAGE
The effects of Rolfing are cumulative. Each session concentrates on a different area of the body, working toward a specific goal.

As a patient you will generally remain passive throughout a session, but the practitioner may ask you occasionally to do something, such as pushing against the Rolfer's hand or stretching a limb, to facilitate the deep massage.

Rolfing was developed during the 1940s by an American biochemist, Dr. Ida Rolf. Originally known as structural integration, the technique involves the manipulation of the fascia—the web of connective tissues that surround the muscles, ligaments, tendons, and internal organs of the body. Wherever the fasciae are shortened or stuck, Rolfing works to lengthen and separate tissues to correct any structural imbalances and achieve realignment of the body. Most people are not aware that their body is out of balance until after it

has been realigned. An example of a person who is unaware of poor posture is one who places most of his or her weight on the heels. This throws the body's center of gravity backward; to compensate, the upper body must tilt forward, thus throwing the pelvis out of alignment. The muscles and the web of fascia that covers them become contracted and stressed in order to hold this unnatural posture. A Rolfer will manipulate the fasciae to disentangle them and thus allow the body to stand vertically at ease within the pull of gravity.

How can Rolfing help me?
Almost everyone has something wrong with his or her posture that Rolfing could improve to allow greater freedom of movement. Aches and pains caused by undue stress placed on muscles and ligaments by poor posture can also be relieved. After a series of treatments, you should have a more upright, relaxed, and centered stature. Movement should be easier and more graceful and be accompanied by increased energy and vitality and improved self-image. Rolfing can also unlock emotional traumas that may be contributing to the way you move and hold yourself.

What happens in the first session?
The Rolfer will first talk through your medical history, asking for details about any existing conditions, such as diabetes or heart disease, accidents, emotional traumas, and

any pain, tension, or discomfort you are currently experiencing. You will then be asked to undress to your underwear. The therapist will take a "before" photograph, which will later be compared with an "after" picture taken following the last session to note postural changes.

The massage takes place with you either lying or sitting on a couch and remaining mostly passive, although you may be asked to make a few simple movements from time to time. During the massage the Rolfer uses fingers, thumbs, hands, and elbows to stretch, separate, and relax the connective tissues.

How long will the treatment last?

Rolfing typically involves a series of 10 sessions spaced 1 to 3 weeks apart, with each session lasting between 60 and 90 minutes. Most Rolfers will allow you to try a session or two to find out whether Rolfing suits you. However, they stress that the benefits of Rolfing are cumulative, and in order to gain the full effect of the therapy, you will need to commit yourself to the entire series. This is because the therapy is structured so that over the complete course each part of the body is worked on progressively.

The first three sessions concentrate on the superficial fasciae around the outer muscles of the body, while the next four focus on the deeper muscles, or the core structure of fasciae. The final three sessions involve integrating all the work so that the muscular system of the body is healed holistically.

Will I find it painful?

Because Rolfing is a deep-tissue massage, it can be uncomfortable or momentarily painful. However, any pain that is felt should be positive, that is, it should be characterized by the feeling of released tension that often accompanies it. The level of discomfort will depend on the individual and how much tension is being held in the body; some people experience no pain at all. Any

discomfort should be bearable, however, and the Rolfer will stop if you request it.

What makes Rolfing different from other body manipulation methods?

The main difference between Rolfing and other body therapies is that Rolfing works the whole body rather than one specific area; it is not geared to treating a particular symptom. Another factor unique to Rolfing is that it may release locked-in emotions. The therapy can be used to aid personal growth and unlock emotional pain. A psychologist may refer someone to a Rolfer for help in releasing trauma on a physical level. Rolfers believe that emotional pain and memories are held not only in the brain but also in the muscle and tissue structure of the body.

Should anyone avoid Rolfing?

Rolfing is suitable for almost anyone, and there are very few contra-indications. However, it is not recommended for people with certain forms of cancer, and it may not be helpful for the severely obese because of the difficulty in reaching the deeper connective tissue.

Recently the technique has proved very successful for repetitive strain injuries, such as carpal tunnel syndrome. Rolfing is compatible with most forms of exercise and sports, although some are contrary to its aims. For example, body building and marathon running involve unnatural posture, which can undo any benefit that has been gained from Rolfing.

What training does a Rolfer have?

A professional Rolfer has been trained by instructors based at the Rolf Institute in Boulder, Colorado. Entrants must meet a minimum requirement in physiology education and should have professionally practiced a hands-on therapy, such as Swedish massage or shiatsu, for at least 200 hours.

WHAT YOU CAN DO AT HOME

A Rolfing treatment usually involves a certain amount of work to do at home, although this will vary from one person to another because individual body structure differs. Sometimes specific exercises or activities may be requested. For example, if someone has a collapsed posture at the front, regular backstroke swimming may help to open up the chest. Certain exercises that concentrate on promoting free breathing, controlled movement, increased flexibility, and improved balance may be recommended to extend the benefits of Rolfing and to enhance the ongoing changes in body structure. Such techniques include Pilates therapy (see page 88), yoga, and t'ai chi.

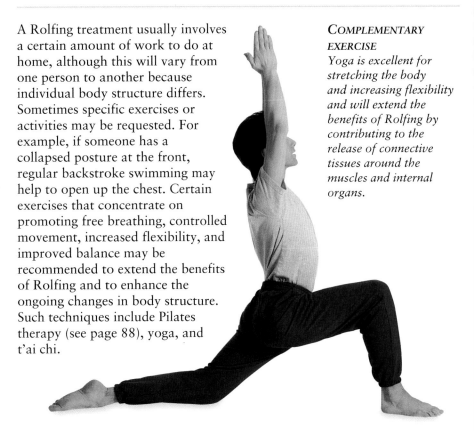

COMPLEMENTARY EXERCISE
Yoga is excellent for stretching the body and increasing flexibility and will extend the benefits of Rolfing by contributing to the release of connective tissues around the muscles and internal organs.

FACTORS THAT AFFECT YOUR SHAPE

Your shape— height, weight, and build—is influenced largely by your sex, age, and genetic inheritance but also to some degree by diet and exercise.

The most important determining factor for your shape is your sex. Apart from the obvious differences between the body shapes of men and women, sex hormones play a major role in dictating how you store fat and the ratio of muscle to fat in your body, affecting to some degree the ease with which you gain or lose weight.

GENDER DIFFERENCES

The male hormone testosterone stimulates bone and muscle growth, as well as male sexual development. At puberty, men experience a growth in muscle bulk and bone size. The most noticeable buildup of muscle mass is in the upper body and arms. By contrast, women become better developed in the leg and hip areas.

Perhaps the most significant difference between men and women in terms of shape, however, lies in the fact that the average man's body fat is about 10 percent lower than a woman's. This difference reflects the fact that a woman's body should carry at least 16 percent fat to maintain proper levels of hormone production and be fertile.

Progesterone, one of the female hormones that governs the reproductive system of women, also causes an increase in the deposition of fat within the body. In addition to promoting the development of breasts and body hair and the onset of menstruation at puberty, female hormones also lead to an increase in body fat around the hips, buttocks, abdomen, and top of the thighs. As women grow older, they tend to store fat not only in those areas but also on their breasts, waist, and the back of the upper arms and shoulders. Men have a tendency to store fat around their abdomen and hips, but they can also store it in other areas.

The skeletal frame of men and women also differs. Men have larger and heavier bones and a narrower pelvic cavity. Relative to her height and build, the average woman has narrower shoulders, a shorter rib cage, and a broader pelvis than a man.

Traditionally, strength has been considered the major physiological difference between men and women, but the gap progressively narrowed between the sexes over the second half of the 20th century. Men still have an advantage in upper body strength because they have proportionally larger lungs and bigger rib cages. However, in terms of lower body muscle strength, women have drawn much closer to men in their abilities. Their performance in this area has improved dramatically over the past 50 years, while men have made only moderate gains during the same period. Currently the best female time for running a marathon, set by Ingrid Kristiansen of

HOW THE GENDERS DIFFER IN BODY SHAPE This young couple illustrates some of the body shape differences between the two sexes. The female has a defined waist and rounded hips. The male is starting to develop muscle bulk in his upper body and arms and has a less defined waist and narrower hips.

Norway, is just a matter of minutes behind the best male time of 2 hours, 6 minutes, and 50 seconds, set by Belayneh Dinsanso of Ethiopia at about the same time.

Some experts estimate that women may run even faster marathons than men within the next 50 years. This indicates the extent to which physical development can be influenced by social norms. Over the past few decades women have begun to challenge their capacity for muscle development and have become enthusiastic participants in previously all-male sports—rugby, football, and bodybuilding, for example.

Despite these areas in which women and men are drawing closer together, women still experience more extensive changes than men in their body shape over a lifetime because they tend to carry more fat than their male counterparts and because their bodies are affected dramatically by pregnancy and menopause.

PREGNANCY

During pregnancy a large number of body changes take place. The body systems of a pregnant woman have great demands made on them, and it is essential to rest, relax, and eat sensibly. During pregnancy calcium is absorbed by the fetus to help build its bones, so a woman must take in adequate calcium to maintain her own reserves. And exercise during pregnancy is as important as at any other stage in life. Regular walking and swimming help keep joints and muscles supple and can be continued right through to the latter stages. Swimming has the additional benefit of supporting the body's weight, which takes the strain off the back and joints. Strenuous or potentially hazardous sports, like running, horseback riding, and skiing, should be avoided.

Backache is a common complaint during pregnancy. This is because the ligaments and fibrous tissue that lock the joints together become more elastic due to hormonal changes. This change allows the pelvis to expand during childbirth, but it also makes the joints in the body vulnerable to strain. This particularly affects the back, which is put under additional strain by having to balance the heavy load of the baby in front.

Many women gain too much weight during pregnancy and then have difficulty in losing it after the birth. A pregnant woman

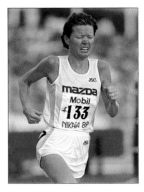

RECORD BREAKER
On April 21, 1985, in the London Marathon, Ingrid Kristiansen recorded the fastest ever marathon time for a woman: 2 hours, 21 minutes, 6 seconds. Just 14 minutes and 16 seconds behind the male record of that time, the result is but one example of the narrowing gap between the athletic abilities of men and women.

WOMEN AND BODYBUILDING

Traditionally a male pursuit, bodybuilding has become popular with women in the past 20 years. This is perhaps evidence of a change in the way that women perceive themselves and what society views as the ideal feminine form. The heavily muscled physiques of female bodybuilders, with their extremely low percentage of body fat and lack of feminine curves, may appear asexual to some. Enthusiasts argue, however, that they reveal the freedom of women to make their own decisions about body image.

Aesthetic preferences aside, there are certain physical disadvantages for women who have such a low percentage of body fat. Their production of the hormones estrogen and progesterone, which trigger ovulation and menstruation, can cease, with possible long-term effects, including infertility and an increased risk of osteoporosis.

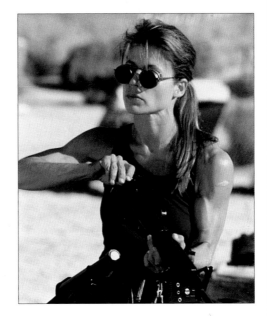

MUSCULAR ATTRACTION
In the film Terminator 2, *Linda Hamilton shows that having muscles does not necessarily diminish female attractiveness.*

Separation of the abdominal muscles

Four sets of muscles surround the abdomen, providing stability for the trunk during movement. A line of thick connective tissue joins these muscles at the midline. As a baby grows during pregnancy, the abdominal muscles are gradually stretched and pushed apart and can separate as a result; this separation is called diastasis recti.

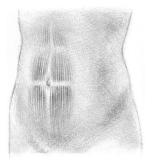

BEFORE PREGNANCY
The abdominal muscles are tightly joined by connective tissue.

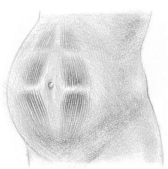

DURING PREGNANCY
The abdominal muscles are stretched apart and may separate.

should gain roughly 20 to 30 pounds. Too much or too little may affect the baby. Also, if less weight is gained, it will be easier to lose any excess after the baby is born.

Once the baby arrives, your obstetritian will recommend specific exercises to help you regain your previous body shape. However, once you recover from the birth, you should also continue other forms of exercise, such as walking and swimming, to maintain joint suppleness and muscle tone. Discuss with your doctor when it is advisable to resume your usual exercise regimen. Usually a fit and healthy mother who had no complications during or after the birth can start exercise classes six to eight weeks after the baby is born, but always check with your medical adviser first.

MENOPAUSE

A woman's monthly periods first begin to diminish and then cease altogether with the onset of menopause, which usually occurs during her late forties to early fifties. Menopause is triggered by the ovaries reducing their production of the female hormone estrogen, and it is this reduced level of estrogen that causes the classic symptoms of the condition, including hot flashes, vaginal

dryness, night sweating, hair and skin changes, chronic fatigue, and in some women, depression.

Lack of estrogen also slows the body's metabolic rate (the rate at which the body uses energy to fuel all physiological functions) but this effect may not manifest itself until a few years later. The lowered metabolism can cause a rise in the level of fats in the blood, and this in turn increases the likelihood of narrowing of the arteries (atherosclerosis) and also the chances of stroke and coronary artery disease.

The effect that menopause has on the bones is one of the most damaging changes. During the first 2 to 5 years after menopause, the bones become thinner; over a period of 10 to 15 years from the onset of menopause, osteoporosis (an increase in the brittleness of the bones) may develop.

Slight weight gain may be experienced, partly because of the slowing of metabolism, but also because as we age we tend to exercise less. A more obvious change that takes place around the time of menopause is in the way that fat is distributed within the body. Before menopause, fat is typically distributed around the buttocks, thighs, and abdomen. After menopause, however, a

---

CORRECTING SEPARATION OF THE ABDOMINAL MUSCLES

Separation of the abdominal muscles can occur during pregnancy when the muscles can stretch no further, though it may not be noticeable during a first pregnancy. Here we show how to check for separation and how to repair the split. The exercise should be performed for 10 repetitions at least 5 times a day. After a week or two, the gap should return to normal—1.25 cm (about ½ inch).

CHECKING FOR SEPARATION
Lie on your back with knees bent and feel down the midline of your abdomen for the gap between your abdominal muscles. If you can fit more than two fingers in the gap, your muscles have separated.

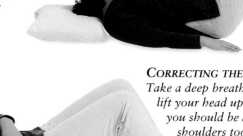

CORRECTING THE SEPARATION
Take a deep breath and, as you exhale, lift your head up (after a few days you should be able to lift your shoulders too). At the same time, gently pull the two sides of the abdominal muscles toward the midline of your stomach. Lie back slowly, then repeat.

OSTEOPOROSIS AND BODY SHAPE

With advancing age, body shape can change due to the effects of osteoporosis, a progressive loss of bone density that results over time in the bones becoming brittle and easily broken. In its severest form the condition causes curvature of the spine, or "dowager's hump," as well as a general loss of height. The vertebrae in the spine may crumble, causing the spine to compress and curve forward. Mild osteoporosis may not cause any ill effects, but the severe form, which is more common in women, can be crippling. Preventive steps include a calcium-rich diet, regular weight-bearing exercise throughout life, and hormone replacement therapy for postmenopausal women.

BONE DENSITY
In healthy bone (below), fibers of the protein collagen provide density and elasticity, while calcium is responsible for hardness. In osteoporitic bone (right), loss of calcium causes brittleness, which can lead to fractures and spinal curvature.

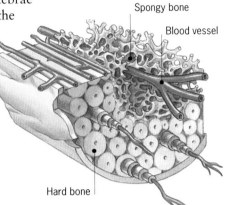

Spongy bone

Blood vessel

Hard bone

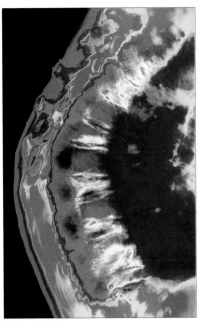

larger proportion of fat tends to be stored around the breasts, waist, lower abdomen, and upper arms. All these body changes are normal, but their effects can be minimized by adjusting your lifestyle to include the right type of exercise. Remember, the earlier you start, the more chance you have of lessening the effects of menopause.

Weight-bearing exercises strengthen both the bones and the muscles, while aerobic exercise strengthens the heart and lungs. Diet is also important. Before age 35 bones are still growing, so a diet that includes enough calcium and vitamin D to metabolize the calcium will help provide you with stronger bones. If you are over 35 years, it is still important to take in sufficient calcium, as this will slow the rate at which bone mass is lost. The current government guideline is an intake of at least 1,500 mg of calcium per day for postmenopausal women and men 65 and older.

AGING AND BODY SHAPE

The aging process has clear effects on the shape of our bodies, although many changes are not inevitable and are as much a result of changes in activities and a more sedentary lifestyle as the aging process itself.

Weight gain seems to be a common feature of aging. Metabolism slows down with age, making it more difficult to lose excess weight. After the age of 30 your metabolic rate declines by approximately 2 percent each decade. The ratio of muscle to fat also alters with age, with a shift in favor of fat. However, the effects of all these changes can be slowed with regular exercise. Recent evidence suggests that the most influential factor in the age-related shape changes is the fact that people become more sedentary as they grow older.

Many people also see frailty and loss of muscle strength as an inevitable effect of aging, but recent research examining the extent to which the elderly can improve their muscle strength through exercise has shown that huge improvements can be made even in old age (see chart, right).

GENETIC INHERITANCE AND ENVIRONMENTAL INFLUENCES

Your body shape is very much dictated by what your parents and grandparents looked like and sometimes even by what an ancient ancestor looked like. This programming is carried in your genes.

Certain predominant characteristics, such as height and build, are handed down through family trees, or genetic inheritance. Genes are contained in chromosomes within a person's body cells. Each chromosome contains a long strand of the hereditary substance deoxyribonucleic acid, or DNA,

STRENGTH IN OLD AGE
A study in 1990 by an American doctor, Maria Fiatarone, showed how exercise can improve the quality of life in old age. After eight weeks of weight training, 10 men and women ages 87 to 96 almost tripled their muscle strength and found they could get around much more easily. Their confidence soared; one man said he felt 50 again!

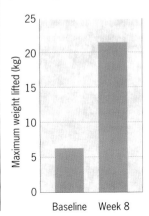

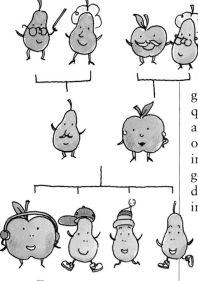

*FAMILY TREE OF
BODY SHAPE
A person's height and
build are believed to be
controlled by the
combined effects of many
genes, along with
environmental effects
that include diet and
exercise. The family tree
shown here consists of
apple- and pear-shaped
people. A child's
tendency toward a
certain shape depends on
the relative number of
genes that determine
body shape passed down
from the parents.*

which transmits all genetic information. When two short people have a child, there is a good chance that the child will also be short because he or she will inherit the genetic tendency to be short from the genetic pools of both parents. However, quantitative characteristics, such as height and skin color, are controlled by a number of different genetic instructions that interact in complex ways. This is known as polygenic inheritance, and its influence makes it difficult to identify a simple pattern of dominant or recessive traits. It is possible, for instance, for two short people to produce a very tall child, depending on the particular interaction of different commands in their genetic blueprints.

Environmental factors, such as quality of health care and nutrition enjoyed by a child, can also influence adult height, although maximum potential size might still be genet-

ically capped at a certain level. Research has shown that as diet improves, children gain in height regardless of their inheritance. This effect can be seen readily in the taller children of immigrants to North America. Another example is found in the height gains measured in children in Great Britain after the Second World War. These were widely attributed to the nutritionally balanced school meals that were made available during the war. Increased intake of calcium has been shown to be particularly important in this regard.

The amount of regular exercise performed during childhood and adolescence also plays a role in encouraging the healthy growth of organs, bones, and muscles. The size of your lungs, for example, is largely determined by the amount of aerobic exercise that you did during adolescence, when your lungs were still developing.

GENES AND HOW THEY AFFECT YOUR SHAPE

Genes are units of hereditary material that are contained in the body's cells. They help to determine all aspects of bodily growth and functioning by directing the manufacture of proteins. All of a person's genes come directly from his or her parents. The genes are contained in a chain of deoxyribonucleic acid, or DNA, which makes up each of

the 46 chromosomes held in every body cell. Each body cell houses this identical structure, or DNA. Everyone has a different DNA pattern, which makes us all distinct individuals with different eye and hair color, body shape, and physical and behavioral characteristics. The only individuals to share the same DNA are identical twins.

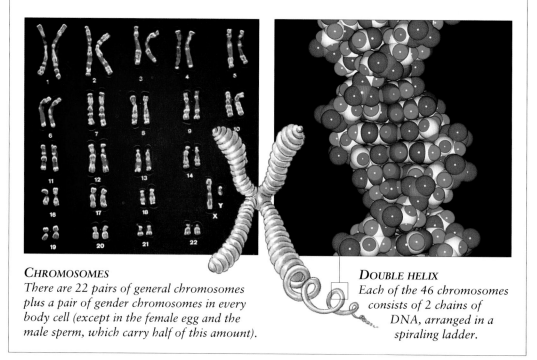

*CHROMOSOMES
There are 22 pairs of general chromosomes plus a pair of gender chromosomes in every body cell (except in the female egg and the male sperm, which carry half of this amount).*

*DOUBLE HELIX
Each of the 46 chromosomes consists of 2 chains of DNA, arranged in a spiraling ladder.*

FAMILY RESEMBLANCE

Visual characteristics can be passed from one generation to the next or can skip a generation, only to reappear later. One famous example is the Hapsburg lip. The Hapsburg dynasty flourished from the 15th to the 19th century, and inter-marriage within the royal houses of Europe produced the striking family trait of a very prominent lower lip. It can be seen in many family portraits. Examples of family resemblances are also evident in the generations of the British royal family. Marriage with other royal families, such as the Romanovs of Russia in the 19th century, has led to some recurring resemblances.

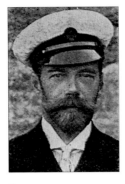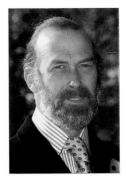

ROYAL LIKENESS
Blood relatives through the female line, Britain's Prince Michael of Kent (right) and Tsar Nicholas II of Russia (left) share family characteristics passed down for centuries.

BODY SHAPE AND RACE

There is a noticeable difference in body shape between people of different races. Anthropologists have many theories about how these variations evolved. One is based on research that has revealed a relationship between the average shape and weight within a group of ethnically related people and the climate in which they live. The colder the weather, for example, the more body fat people tend to carry. A rounded, short-limbed body shape conserves heat more efficiently, and this shape is predominant in the Arctic regions (see photograph, below right).

The most efficient way to lose heat from the body is to have an extended surface area from which to lose it; accordingly, people who live in the desert, such as the Australian aborigines and many African tribes, have long, slender arms and legs.

Body shape is also governed by diet. Anthropologists believe that the bodies of people who live in poorly nourished countries gradually changed to ensure their survival. In an area ranging from Egypt to India, southern China, and Southeast Asia, a body shape developed that is small and slight. This is because the smaller the body, the fewer calories it requires for survival. As the bodies of people living in this wide area became progressively smaller, it meant that they could produce more work on a smaller and smaller intake of calories. In contrast, countries like Australia and New Zealand have tall populations. This is partly because of intermarriage between different types of

people, but the increase in height of individuals who are from a traditionally short Celtic-Irish background has been attributed to the high-protein and high-calcium diet typical of these countries.

Many variations on these broad principles occur, governed by the human ability to modify diet and the environment by growing certain food plants and animals and by building shelters as protection from the elements. These adaptations enable people of the "wrong" shape to live successfully in hostile environments.

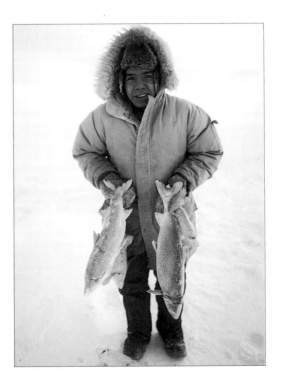

KEEPING WARM IN THE ARCTIC
Indigenous to the Arctic region, the Inuits are a good example of how human body shape has adapted to the environment. Their characteristically short and squat bodies conserve energy efficiently. Traditionally, the Inuits wore animal skins to keep themselves warm. Today, however, clothing made with such fabrics as Gore-Tex and Polartec keeps out the elements and helps visitors from other climates keep warm as well.

PERCEPTIONS OF NORMAL SHAPE

Before you begin a shaping-up program, it may be helpful to think about how much your perception of an ideal shape might be influenced by unrealistic dictates of fashion and society.

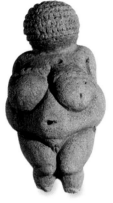

VENUS OF WILLENDORF
This ancient sandstone sculpture dates from the Paleolithic period around 20,000 B.C. The very full figure is believed to celebrate the beauty of the fertile female form.

SHAPE AND POWER
The wealth and status of King Henry VIII was conveyed by his imposing figure. At a time when malnutrition posed a real threat to large numbers of ordinary people, Henry continued to gain weight, symbolizing his own personal prosperity throughout his reign.

Throughout the ages the "acceptable" shape for women and, to a lesser degree, men has varied, and people have always responded to the fashions of their day. The chances are quite random that any person's natural body shape happens to be fashionable, and yet people go to great lengths to try to achieve a shape that contradicts their genetic inheritance if that is what fashion demands.

CHANGES THROUGHOUT HISTORY
Although today Western society associates attractiveness with being slim, thin has not always been in fashion. From the time of ancient cultures until the 19th century, plump was associated with a woman's fertility, and until the latter part of the 20th century, fertility was greatly valued. Neolithic fertility goddesses were round bellied,

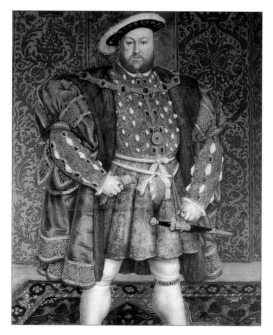

wide hipped, and full breasted, reflecting the ideal woman to ensure a man's genetic line. The worship of mother figures continued with the adoration of the Madonna, and Renaissance paintings of the Virgin focused on the breasts and belly without actually depicting any flesh; her modesty was protected with generous swaths of cloth.

Fat was not associated solely with women and fertility; it also indicated a person's wealth and status. The rich could afford to eat more and were less likely to perform any physical activity. Similarly, courtesans of the courts of Europe for much of the past three centuries were large, plump women who were lazy, indolent, and given to hedonism.

For men there has been pressure throughout the centuries to present a manly figure. Doublet and hose revealed quite an expanse of male leg from the 14th century onward, hemlines of tunics rising so high that by the mid-15th century, modesty dictated the need for a codpiece (a flap that concealed the opening in the breeches). Occasionally men used padding and binding to improve on nature. It was not uncommon for 18th-century beaux to use padding on their calves.

While being thin may have become fashionable in relatively recent times, manipulating shapes to exaggerate the narrowness of a woman's waist in relation to her bust and hips has had a long tradition. Some theorists argue that this is because men are genetically programmed to associate a good waist-hip ratio with fertility; in the interests of protecting their genetic line, they have an eye for childbearing hips indicated by a slim waist. To achieve this look, corsetry was used for centuries; in the Victorian and Edwardian eras, a tiny waist was accompanied first by crinolines and then the bustle

FASHION AND THE IDEAL BODY SHAPE

Today's fashion industry is often blamed for contributing to the rise of eating disorders, such as anorexia nervosa and bulimia, as people strive to be as thin as fashion models. But fashion has dictated body shape and defined sexuality for many centuries, and the "ideal" shape of the moment has always had a powerful effect. Some Edwardian women, for example, had their lower ribs surgically removed so that their corsets could be pulled tighter to achieve the hourglass figure fashionable at the time.

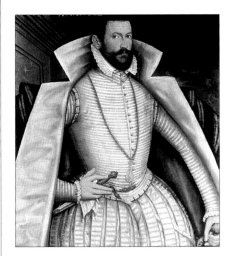

ELIZABETHAN ÉLAN
Elizabethan men were as figure conscious as women. Corsets were used to reduce their waists, with pantaloons exaggerating the effect.

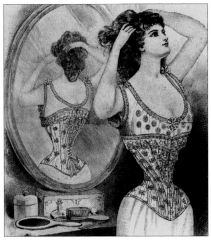

EDWARDIAN CORSETRY
Edwardian fashion demanded impossibly petite waists, achievable only with heavy corsetry that distorted the spine and compressed the stomach.

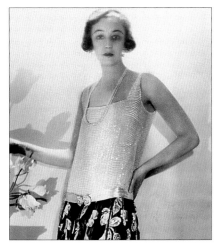

1920S MINIMALISM
The fashionable body shape for women in the 1920s was slim and boyish. Clothes skimmed waists and breasts were bound to achieve a flat chest.

to exaggerate the hips and buttocks. Such a physique was so unnatural that it could be achieved only with the aid of tightly laced corsets. The appeal of this fashion was so great that some Edwardian men also adopted corsets to achieve a slimmer waist. For both women and men, tight lacing dangerously compressed the abdominal organs and made breathing labored. Exercise was uncomfortable, but then, only the most moderate of exertion was considered genteel.

At the end of World War I, when women got the vote, their new freedom was reflected in their dress. The flapper look allowed free movement, and skirts rose daringly to the knee, revealing women's legs for the first time in history. The fashionable body shape of the time was flat chested, so women began dieting and binding their breasts to make them look smaller. In the young upper-class set, it became fashionable to take drugs to achieve a slim figure, a trend that continued throughout the following decades.

After World War II there was a widespread push initially toward a return to traditional values. Women were encouraged by government policy to leave the workforce and return to their traditional role as homemaker and mother. They were expected to remain at home while their husbands went out and worked to support the family. Christian Dior's "new look" in many ways emphasized a womanly figure, with full skirts that exaggerated the width of the hips and very structured conical-shaped bras that pushed the breasts forward. Nipped waistlines exaggerated curves further still. At the same time the male role as provider and protector was emphasized by wide-shouldered suits that gave an impression of both strength and power.

Another revolution occurred in the 1960s with the arrival of the miniskirt. It was during this period that female attractiveness became firmly linked with youth. Motherhood was out of fashion, and society was inspired by the culture of youth; models like Twiggy set a new vogue for thin, boyish figures. Designers followed suit with shapeless shift dresses that disguised natural female curves. Fashion for men also started to focus on boyish shapes. The "mod" look,

SYMPTOMS OF ANOREXIA

There are a number of behavioral and physical indicators that indicate anorexia. These are

▶ *rapid and very noticeable weight loss—ranging from 25 to 33 percent of the person's normal weight*

▶ *hyperactivity*

▶ *obsessive exercising*

▶ *preoccupation with food*

▶ *unwillingness to eat in company*

▶ *hiding food*

▶ *inability to sleep*

▶ *disruption or cessation of the menstrual cycle*

▶ *an increase in the density of the soft coating of hair that covers the skin*

with its drainpipe jeans and tight-fitting shirts, was designed for the thin, boyish figures of pop stars like Roger Daltry.

Although today we may think we have a more balanced view about appearance, there is still plenty of evidence that we often go to extremes to achieve an ideal shape. Slimness is still the order of the day, but with the added pressure on women to have curves in the right places. Eating disorders appear to be increasing among both sexes, while cosmetic surgery has recently become a popular option for both men and women who are unhappy with their shape. (Although there are surgical options for altering body shape, any decision to undergo such surgery should be well researched and thought through.)

DISTORTED SHAPE PERCEPTION

At some stage most of us would like to change aspects of our shape, but for some people shape is a dangerous obsession. A lack of self-confidence and self-esteem can lead to focusing on shape as the solution to a person's unhappiness. In extreme cases the eating disorders anorexia and bulimia can develop. These psychologically based illnesses can cause severe physical problems. Sufferers, who have a terror of putting on weight, possess a very distorted view of their bodies—even at their most gaunt they believe they are fat and ugly. Such a negative self-image and desire for an unrealistic body shape cause such distress that feelings

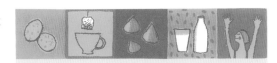

SUPER SHAPER

It is a myth that potatoes are fattening. In fact, they are mostly carbohydrate, which is an energy food with less than half the calories of fat. It is the oil or fat used to cook potatoes or that is added as a topping that makes them fattening. Potatoes also contain protein and fiber and are good sources of potassium and vitamin C. For healthier eating, avoid french-fried potatoes and chips and opt for boiled or baked versions. Most of the fiber and nutrients are in the skin, so they are best when eaten unpeeled.

of self-loathing dominate. Various behavioral patterns accompany eating disorders. These include a tendency toward compulsiveness and perfection, as well as a fear of sexual development. Although in a few cases there may be a possible genetic or metabolic cause, society's promotion of thinness as attractive is thought to play a very significant role.

Little is known about why certain people develop eating disorders, although there are some clues provided by its tendency to occur in specific sections of society. Usually the sufferers are young, female, white, and

THE RISKS OF COSMETIC BREAST SURGERY

It is common for women to be dissatisfied with the size and shape of their breasts, no matter what kind of figure they have. Some women feel so strongly that they choose to undergo cosmetic surgery.

A breast enlargement, reduction, or lift should not be undertaken lightly or without a complete understanding of the risks. All procedures are likely to involve some degree of scarring and also carry the risk of infection, breast pain, loss of sensation, and complications for breast-feeding. Implants may move, leak, or make the breasts feel unnaturally firm a few years after the operation. Leakage is a familiar complication of silicone

implants. A suspected link with cancer led to a ban of these implants in the United States, but recent studies suggest that any risk is so low as to be negligible. Other studies have linked silicone leakage with the development of autoimmune disorders, but these findings are also controversial, with many health professionals denying any such link.

A more direct danger may be that silicone implants mask the presence of tumors or cysts on mammograms, possibly allowing a developing cancer to go undetected. Women who have a family history of breast cancer should therefore avoid silicone implants.

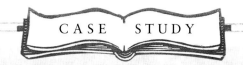

A Self-Obsessed Woman

People who are overly preoccupied with their body shape and weight often have an underlying sense of inadequacy. Controlling their bodies may make them feel that they have more power over their lives, but taken to an extreme, this tunnel-visioned effort toward perfection can take away all pleasure, fuel insecurities, and place excessive pressures on body and mind.

Jill is an ambitious 35-year-old sales manager. She has a lot of drive and works long hours building up her client list. Her staff finds her demanding and notices her absence at social gatherings. Jill goes to the gym every night, where she is just as demanding of herself physically as she is professionally. Jill is intelligent and attractive, but finds it hard to start a relationship and often feels lonely. She doesn't tell people about her problems because she appears so successful. During a weekend visit with Pam, an old school friend, Jill confessed how unhappy she was. Pam advised her to stop being so hard on herself and those around her. Jill found this recommendation difficult to accept but promised Pam she would think about it.

What should Jill do?

Jill needs to accept that she is pushing herself too hard and that the expectations she believes she has to live up to are only her own. Her need to control herself and everyone around her is narrowing her life, and her demanding physical workouts are a symptom of her driving need for perfection. If she relinquishes some control, her life will open up of its own accord.

Jill needs to talk with someone about how she is feeling and decide on some areas that she can change. She should avoid going to the gym so much that she works herself to exhaustion. She could investigate ways of exercising that might be less intense and start saying yes to social invitations.

WORK
Making working life enjoyable for others is part of being a good manager. Work is important, but it is only one part of life.

FITNESS
Using exercise as a means of control can be dangerous. Never push yourself to reach unachievable goals.

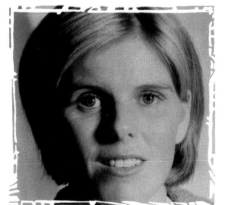

EMOTIONAL HEALTH
Making yourself physically perfect won't automatically lead to a fulfilling life.

Action Plan

WORK
Try to develop a more relaxed attitude toward work goals and focus on team-building and cooperation as a means to achieving them.

FITNESS
Cut down on gym visits and work-out lengths. Look at more sociable ways to exercise; join a sport team or walking group, for example.

EMOTIONAL HEALTH
Life shouldn't be all work and no play. Make some time to build a social network and relate to people on an emotional level.

How things turned out for Jill

Jill began to realize she was obsessive and felt relief once she acknowledged that she didn't have to outperform everyone. Her change in attitude made her more open, and people at work began to notice that she was more relaxed and willing to give rather than demand. She also began to focus more on her personal relationships and she joined the company softball team, which is paying off in a more enjoyable social life.

STEPS TO IMPROVE SELF-IMAGE

A positive self-image is important for everyone. Insecurities about looks are often unfounded but can still leave a person feeling miserable and inadequate. Following the steps below can help you achieve satisfaction with your body.

▶ *Work out your BMI (see page 16); you may find that your weight is actually healthy.*

▶ *Buy clothes that flatter your shape and disguise problem areas (see Chapter 3).*

▶ *Exercise regularly. Exercise releases endorphins, which help lift your mood.*

▶ *Don't put yourself in a situation that makes you feel inadequate. If you are the only overweight person in an aerobics class full of the superfit, change classes.*

middle class. It is estimated that approximately 1 in every 100 people in this group suffers an eating disorder. This figure rises to a ratio of 1 in 20 among those who use their bodies in their profession—dancers, models, actresses, and female athletes.

Although there are numerous theories about the psychological aspects of eating disorders, doctors, nutritionists, and often the sufferers themselves cannot truly say why they have such an unhappy relationship with food and their bodies.

Anyone who suffers an eating disorder must seek professional help. Left untreated, it can cause severe damage to the body; in the worst cases death may occur through starvation. The first line of attack is often a course of antidepressants followed by counseling and/or psychotherapy. The underlying psychological factors are explored and nutritional supervision provided to reeducate the sufferer in better eating habits. These treatments may last for several years. Severe cases often require hospitalization for a time and supervised convalescence.

Recovery from an eating disorder is a long, slow, and not always permanent process. There are a few alternative therapies that can be useful in supporting a sufferer's medical care. Hypnotherapy can help to identify the causes of the distorted self-image; autosuggestion can nurture a more positive view about body shape and size; and acupuncture can help to relieve stress and rebalance the body's energy.

FEELING GOOD ABOUT YOUR BODY SHAPE

While anorexia and bulimia are relatively rare illnesses, emotional fixations on weight and shape are common. Numerous studies have revealed the extent to which people's sense of self-worth is dangerously linked to their appearance. Feeling good about your appearance does contribute to self-confidence, but your view of your shape should be kept in perspective. No one is exclusively defined by appearance; personality, intelligence, outlook, behavior, and beliefs all contribute to who you are.

SHAPING UP AND THE IDEAL BODY

It is important to keep your shaping-up goals realistic and not be influenced by the media's portrayal of an "ideal" shape that may not be healthy for you. Being thin doesn't mean you are healthy; in fact, having too small an amount of body fat can put your health at risk. A lot can be achieved through a carefully planned shaping-up program, but it is vital to keep your focus on good health.

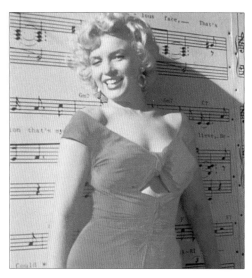

MARILYN MONROE
Whether or not womanly curves are considered fashionable, Marilyn's sex appeal remains constant.

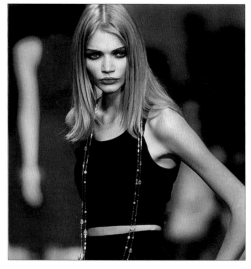

JODIE KIDD
Personifying the waif look of the 1990s fashion world, model Jodie Kidd has been accused of being anorexic.

CHAPTER 2

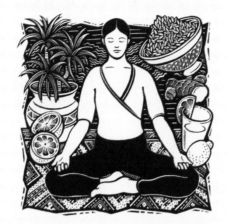

READING YOUR BODY SHAPE

Your body is in many ways a physical record of the psychological and emotional stresses that you experience during life. Reading your shape can provide vital information about your attitudes and major methods of coping. This chapter looks at a range of body-reading therapies and how they can reveal and address underlying tensions that hinder the development of healthy posture and shape.

BODY READING

Body-reading techniques, used in both Eastern and Western therapies, play an important part in revealing emotional, psychological, and physical problems that need to be addressed.

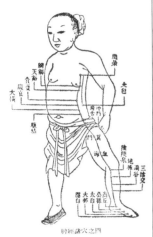

ENERGY MERIDIANS
This Chinese drawing depicts one of the main meridian lines used in acupuncture. It is believed that chi, or life energy, flows along these paths and that its free, unrestricted flow is vital for an aligned and centered body.

CLASS PRESSURE
These students are too intent on their exam papers to worry about the well-being of their backs as they write. Schools tend to do little to encourage good posture while students are working. As can be seen here, saving space is often given priority in classroom design.

At birth you enter the world programmed with a basic shape derived from the genetic blueprint inherited from your parents. In a small percentage of cases, genetic or developmental abnormalities occur, but in most instances an infant's physique is as unblemished as it is ever going to be. Throughout life this basic form will be reshaped by a variety of physical forces that act upon it, like injury, disease, and diet, as well as exercise habits, current fashions, and such occupational factors as working in a physically demanding job. Some psychological and emotional factors play an important part in shaping your physical form too. Tension is a major contributor, but inner conflicts will also be mirrored in your outward appearance.

The ability to gauge a person's psychological and emotional state of health from a study of physical shape is called body reading, and it is a vital component of many Eastern therapies, such as Tuina, t'ai chi, and shiatsu. Body reading is also important in many complementary health therapies

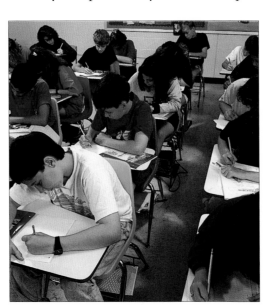

that have developed in the West, such as Rolfing, chiropractic, osteopathy, bioenergetics, and neo-Reichian therapy.

STRESS AND THE BODY
Your body reflects your emotional state, mental attitude, and physical condition through the way you sit, stand, and move around. When you are happy, for example, your mood is mirrored in freer, bouncier movements and a more erect posture. When you are sad or withdrawn, it is shown in a more compressed stance and stiff movements. Physical changes are clearly evident in reaction to stress. Acute stress—brought on by injury, accident, or tragic news, for instance—will immediately shake your emotional makeup and affect your posture. Slumped shoulders, a downcast expression, and weak knees are common reactions.

Long-term unresolved stress, such as ongoing work or relationship problems, often has a more subtle effect. This is because the postures and facial expressions you adopt are designed to mask your inner turmoil so that you can carry on your daily life without drawing attention to your true feelings. Many common expressions reflect this attempt to cope with inner tension: gritting teeth, presenting a fixed smile, and carrying the weight of the world on the shoulders.

Constant tension affects various parts of the body in different ways. The face becomes tight and fairly expressionless as the muscles of the mouth, jaw, and eyes stiffen up to hide emotions; the back becomes rigid as the muscles lose flexibility; the head drops forward, putting an uneven load on the neck, which can no longer keep the head balanced easily; and the shoulders become tense and rounded.

Tension can also cause the pelvis to slump forward, putting the spine out of alignment and exaggerating the appearance of any

AREAS OF TENSION IN THE BODY

The buildup of tension within the body can be caused by many different aspects of a person's life. Occupational influences, such as working at a computer or constantly lifting things;

emotional factors, like a difficult relationship; and psychological factors, such as lack of confidence, all create stress. Tension builds up between major body parts, resulting in tight bands of muscle that fragment the unity of the body.

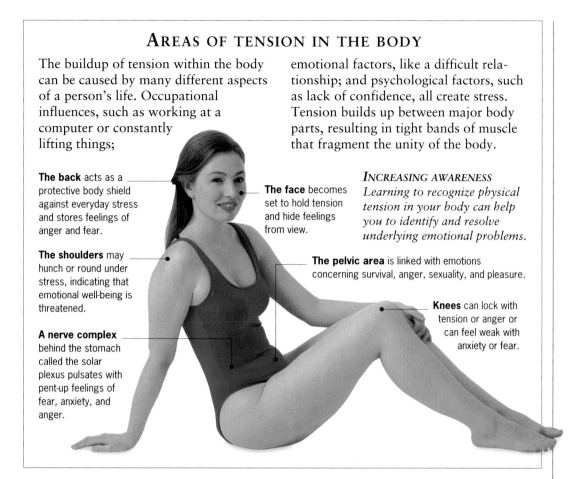

The back acts as a protective body shield against everyday stress and stores feelings of anger and fear.

The shoulders may hunch or round under stress, indicating that emotional well-being is threatened.

A nerve complex behind the stomach called the solar plexus pulsates with pent-up feelings of fear, anxiety, and anger.

The face becomes set to hold tension and hide feelings from view.

INCREASING AWARENESS
Learning to recognize physical tension in your body can help you to identify and resolve underlying emotional problems.

The pelvic area is linked with emotions concerning survival, anger, sexuality, and pleasure.

Knees can lock with tension or anger or can feel weak with anxiety or fear.

surplus flesh around the abdominal area. The legs become stiffer and less flexible, which in turn affects balance and creates an unnaturally rigid gait, counteracting the body's natural flowing movements. Chronic tension is a contributing factor in many physical disorders, including backache, neckache, myalgic facial pain, migraines and other headaches, indigestion, stomach ulcers, joint ailments, breathing disorders, and heart problems.

READING YOUR BODY
Body reading provides a reference system that you can use to evaluate your physical form. Habitual ways of standing that reflect your basic persona can become firmly entrenched. By learning to read these signs, you can judge whether there are deep-seated aspects of your emotional life or psychological profile that you might need to tackle. Subtle abnormalities that might indicate problems are hard to spot in others, but by becoming more familiar with your own body, you can learn to recognize areas that seem to be out of alignment, underdeveloped, or abnormally compacted.

In order to read your body from all angles, you will need a full-length mirror and a handheld one or two large mirrors. Choose a time when you are feeling relaxed. Stand naked in front of the mirror with your back straight and head erect to try to gain an overall impression of your body, then look at each part of it in turn.

Asymmetries and splits
One important aspect of body reading is the ability to identify asymmetries in the body's overall shape. No one is truly symmetrical. Features on one side of the face will differ marginally from those on the other side, for instance, and your dominant arm is likely to be more developed than the other. A pronounced asymmetry, however, such as a steeper slope to one shoulder or a marked tilt to the hips, may indicate a postural fault or musculoskeletal disorder that could lead to serious physical problems.

If half of the body seems out of proportion compared to the other half, it is called a split. A left/right split occurs when all of one side seems noticeably more muscular or better defined than the other, for example,

EYE ASYMMETRY
No one is truly symmetrical, and facial asymmetry is common, particularly around the eyes. On this face the left eye appears more open, outgoing, and receptive, while the right eye looks more tense, closed, and defensive.

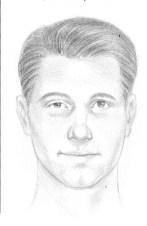

35

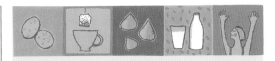

SUPER SHAPER

Herbal teas present a healthy alternative to tea and coffee. There are many types available, and some have beneficial properties; for example, chamomile promotes relaxation and lemon invigorates.

Although caffeine gives an initial energy boost and can relieve fatigue in the short term, in large amounts (over five cups of tea, coffee, or cola drinks a day) it can actually cause fatigue. And in people who suffer anxiety, caffeine can increase anxiety and depression, therefore adding to tension held in the body. Also, a recent study in the Netherlands found that people who drank six cups of unfiltered coffee a day had increased blood levels of homocysteine and cholesterol, both associated with a higher risk of heart disease.

or softer and more rounded. This configuration may indicate inner conflict between the dominant and passive sides of your nature.

A top/bottom split is closely linked with sexual development. In general, men have broad shoulders and narrow hips, and women have the opposite characteristics. A pronounced split is indicated when, allowing for gender differences, the body seems top- or bottom-heavy. Top-heavy people tend to be dominating and aggressive, whereas bottom-heavy people are often seen as passive and unassertive.

In a front/back split, the impression created by your front view seems at variance with the back view. For example, your front, which represents the image you wish to show to the world, may seem angular, muscular, and well defined, while the back view, representing your hidden feelings, may appear softer, weaker, and more vulnerable.

Reading individual body parts

Individual parts of the body also reveal a lot about your emotional profile. Although the face changes expression constantly, certain entrenched characteristics tend to stand out. For example, the eyes may be naturally large and friendly or small and defensive. Sometimes there is a left/right split, indicating mixed inner feelings. The mouth may be full and relaxed or thin and tense. Tension may be seen in a clenched jaw or furrowed brow. The jaw may thrust forward, showing aggression or determination, or recede, thus indicating submission.

HOW YOUR PERSONALITY AFFECTS YOUR BODY

Your personality plays a significant part in your shape, posture, stance, and movement—in short, your body profile. To understand these influences, you need to make an objective assessment of your personality. Study the body profiles to the right to see if you recognize any traits of your own. You may identify with more than one.

To make permanent changes to your body profile, you have to change your behavior. If you recognize any problem areas in your personality, look at the guidelines for change. Change doesn't happen overnight and may be difficult, but just accepting your weaknesses is a big step in the right direction.

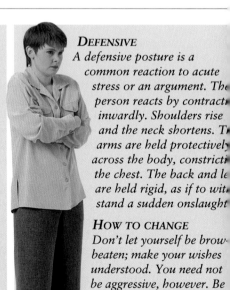

STOICAL
The stoic posture is seen in people who are under constant stress. As if bearing a heavy burden, their bodies look compressed, with a shortened neck, short torso, and stooped shoulders. In addition, their pelvis is tilted forward and their leg muscles are compacted.

HOW TO CHANGE
You do not have to put up with everything in life. Be prepared to rebel from time to time. When people expect you to put yourself out, do not be afraid to say no. State your objections clearly, and people will respect you for it.

DEFENSIVE
A defensive posture is a common reaction to acute stress or an argument. The person reacts by contractr inwardly. Shoulders rise and the neck shortens. Tr arms are held protectively across the body, constricti the chest. The back and le are held rigid, as if to witr stand a sudden onslaught

HOW TO CHANGE
Don't let yourself be brow-beaten; make your wishes understood. You need not be aggressive, however. Be patient while the other pers makes his or her case, and then state yours. Withdraw a discussion becomes heater

The position of the head and neck provides a clear signal of psychological and emotional states. An erect, forward-angled head may suggest competitiveness, assertiveness, and even aggression, especially if accompanied by a jutting jaw. If the head is downcast, however, it may indicate submission or depression. A head held upright appears confident and resolute, whereas a head held back may reflect stubbornness or defensiveness. If the head is tilted to one side, it can suggest indecision or lack of commitment.

The shoulders and arms may be held back in a way that suggests determination, or pushed forward in a protective posture. Raised shoulders indicate a naturally defensive stance, while drooping shoulders may suggest an acceptance of defeat.

The shape of your chest is determined by your normal breathing pattern and indirectly reflects your psychological profile. An over-inflated chest suggests an outwardly dominant and competitive persona. This might, however, be masking a deep-seated sense of insecurity. A sunken chest may indicate a passive or even defensive person who is unable to let go emotionally.

In Eastern cultures the abdomen is seen as the seat of the emotions and is thought to be an important indicator of inner feelings. The abdominal area is also important in body reading for other reasons. The abdominal muscles play a part in all major movements of the upper body, and general tensions or imbalances in the torso will be reflected there, perhaps in a tense and rigid abdomen. The abdominal area is also where excess fat due to overeating is most likely to be deposited and thus may indicate a more general psychological malaise in which food is an important compensation.

The buttocks and pelvis are associated with sexual feelings. A vertical pelvis with firm but relaxed buttock muscles ensures relaxed and free-flowing movement and reflects a well-balanced temperament. A pelvis that is tilted forward combined with loose buttock muscles may indicate weakness and passivity, and a backward-tilted pelvis and tight buttocks may indicate tension and pent-up emotions.

The legs are important indicators of physical and psychological health. Ideally, they should be straight, strong, flexible, and evenly balanced to support the body and produce easy, flowing movements. A knock-kneed stance can indicate insecurity, and legs kept protectively together make mobility slow and awkward. A bow-legged stance suggests imbalance and uncertainty, making movement more unsteady.

continued on page 40

USING BODY LANGUAGE

Your body language can let you down in important situations, such as interviews and business meetings. Here are some tips on how to appear open and receptive:

▶ *To convey confidence, hold your head upright with a relaxed jaw. Try to make eye contact as much as you can during the meeting.*

▶ *Don't cross your arms because this can make you appear defensive.*

▶ *Sit tall with your feet firmly on the floor and your shoulders back and relaxed. When engaged in conversation, lean toward the other person to show your interest.*

▶ *Avoid fidgeting or you will appear nervous.*

▶ *Remember to smile.*

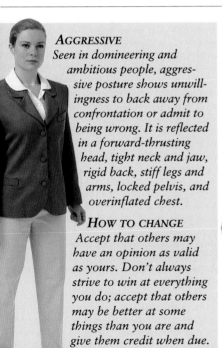

AGGRESSIVE
Seen in domineering and ambitious people, aggressive posture shows unwillingness to back away from confrontation or admit to being wrong. It is reflected in a forward-thrusting head, tight neck and jaw, rigid back, stiff legs and arms, locked pelvis, and overinflated chest.

HOW TO CHANGE
Accept that others may have an opinion as valid as yours. Don't always strive to win at everything you do; accept that others may be better at some things than you are and give them credit when due.

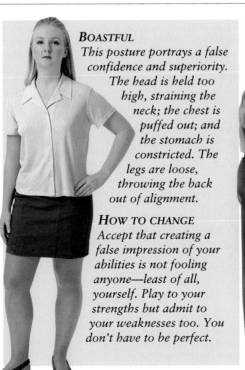

BOASTFUL
This posture portrays a false confidence and superiority. The head is held too high, straining the neck; the chest is puffed out; and the stomach is constricted. The legs are loose, throwing the back out of alignment.

HOW TO CHANGE
Accept that creating a false impression of your abilities is not fooling anyone—least of all, yourself. Play to your strengths but admit to your weaknesses too. You don't have to be perfect.

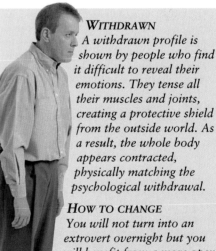

WITHDRAWN
A withdrawn profile is shown by people who find it difficult to reveal their emotions. They tense all their muscles and joints, creating a protective shield from the outside world. As a result, the whole body appears contracted, physically matching the psychological withdrawal.

HOW TO CHANGE
You will not turn into an extrovert overnight but you will benefit from a more open attitude. Be interested in what others are doing. If you make the first move in starting a friendly conversation, you will find it is quickly reciprocated.

The Tuina Practitioner

Tuina is a vigorous physical therapy that is used to relieve the buildup of tension in your body and to treat illness and injury. It can also reveal and help to release emotional factors that may lie behind physical symptoms.

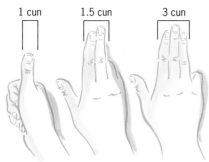

MEASURING CHI POINTS
The cun is a unit used in Chinese medicine to measure the distance of chi points from the bones and muscles of the body.

Literally meaning "push grasp," Tuina is a massage therapy that has been practiced in China for about 4,000 years. Today it is an integral part of the medicinal practices of China. Tuina is a physical therapy involving deep, invigorating massage to release blocked chi, or life energy. In Chinese medical theory this energy flows through channels in the body known as meridians. A practitioner of Tuina exerts pressure along these meridians and at specific points—known as chi points—to release any blockages and enable the

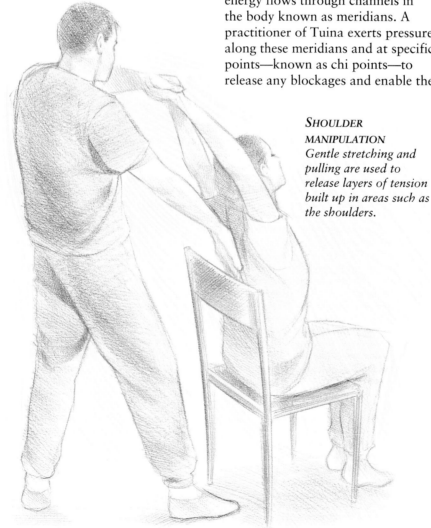

SHOULDER MANIPULATION
Gentle stretching and pulling are used to release layers of tension built up in areas such as the shoulders.

chi to flow through the body unhindered. The free distribution of this energy is thought to have enormous effects on a person's well-being—physically, emotionally, intellectually, and spiritually. A Tuina massage session releases not only the energy of the patient but also that of the therapist. This mutual releasing and exchanging of chi is believed to be beneficial to both participants.

How do I find a Tuina therapist?

Tuina is still emerging as a therapy in the West, but there is a growing number of fully trained therapists. You can find a Tuina practitioner by calling an acupuncture college or contacting the American Oriental Bodywork Association on the Internet. Because Tuina involves a vigorous massage, your therapist should be fully qualified.

Who can benefit from Tuina?

In China, Tuina massage is used as a therapy from the age of five upward. The therapy consists of deep massage but is used in varying intensities on different people. For example, the same depth of massage would not be used on an elderly person as on a younger one. Infants under five are not believed to have fully developed meridian systems, so the therapy is concentrated on the feet and hands in very young children.

Tuina should not be received by anyone with serious heart disease, cancer (especially of the skin or lymphatic system), fractures, lesions, wounds, phlebitis, an infection, or osteoporosis. It can be adapted during pregnancy but should not be applied to the lower abdomen.

Is it a safe therapy?
Tuina is considered very safe, although there may be some bruising in susceptible people. If the wrong point on a meridian is stimulated, no benefit will be gained by the patient but no harm will be done either; the chi will soon rebalance itself if it is stimulated incorrectly.

What sort of problems can Tuina help treat?
Tuina is especially good for treating musculoskeletal problems, sports injuries, and muscular aches. It can also be used to relieve the symptoms of stress-related disorders and such ailments as asthma, migraine, and irritable bowel syndrome. It is not used as a mild, relaxing massage.

Traditional Chinese medicine, of which Tuina is a part, is primarily concerned with preventing disease, but it treats chronic conditions as well. Chinese medical philosophy sees the progress from health to illness as a journey along which symptoms like dizziness or nausea can be observed. Tuina or acupuncture is used to maintain general good health and to check serious ailments before they have a chance to take hold.

How will a consultation start?
Tuina massage is a holistic therapy that works to benefit your entire body and mind. The therapist will begin by asking you questions about your current state of health and mind and your lifestyle. From this point he or she will draw conclusions about which meridian lines need to be worked on during the therapy and, more specifically, at which points on the meridians the energy may be blocked. It is essential to feel relaxed with the practitioner; communication is important throughout the massage session.

What is involved during a Tuina massage?
A Tuina session usually lasts for 30 minutes to an hour. The client wears loose clothing but no shoes. A whole-body massage may begin with a seated neck and shoulder massage, then the practitioner will ask you to move to a massage table or floor mat. The focus of attention is usually on sites where there is pain, meridians, acupressure points, and stiff muscles and joints.

Sometimes heavy pressure is used, which may feel uncomfortable at first, especially if the muscles are particularly tense. The practitioner will usually start with gentler pressure and progress to a deeper and more vigorous massage as your body relaxes. The manipulations should never cause intense pain, however, and if they do, you should tell the therapist immediately.

How will I feel afterward?
On the whole, most people feel revitalized and energetic after a Tuina treatment. Because the therapy releases any blocked emotional energy when the flow of chi is stimulated, however, you may be surprised to find yourself close to tears or feeling excessively emotional after a treatment. This could even occur a few hours or a couple of days later. If this happens, the Chinese approach to dealing with such emotion is to acknowledge its presence and then release it. This release of feelings is good for your emotional health and well-being.

WHAT YOU CAN DO AT HOME

It is easy to incorporate a Tuina self-massage into your daily routine. Find a place to relax and make sure your clothing is loose and comfortable. The room should be warm and softly lit because bright lights may prevent your eyes from relaxing.

Start by using your right hand, clenched in a loose fist, to pummel the outside of your left arm up to the shoulder and down the inside. Repeat this procedure several times and then switch to the other arm. Next, support your right elbow with your left hand and reach over your shoulder to pummel your upper back. Reach back as far as you can. Repeat this procedure with the left arm supported by your right hand. Continue for about a minute, even longer if you prefer. Your upper back should feel relaxed and tingling.

Next, pummel the front of your chest, especially your rib cage, using both hands and continuing for at least a minute. Then bend forward from a standing position and pummel down both sides of your back and buttocks. Using the heels of your hands, vigorously rub the center of your lower back in the area where your kidneys are. Remaining in this forward-leaning position, move your legs apart and pummel down the outside and then the inside of both legs simultaneously.

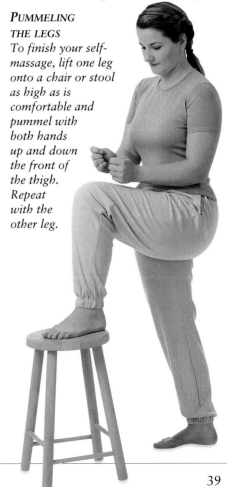

PUMMELING THE LEGS
To finish your self-massage, lift one leg onto a chair or stool as high as is comfortable and pummel with both hands up and down the front of the thigh. Repeat with the other leg.

The feet are very important in Eastern body reading because they allow energy to flow through the body and provide contact with the earth. This contact is called grounding. In grounded people the foot is supple and keeps the body balanced by ensuring that the weight is evenly distributed. In ungrounded people the foot is weak and flat or rigid and excessively arched, leaving them unbalanced, unsteady, and slow to react.

PRACTICAL STEPS TO CHANGING YOUR BODY PROFILE

Once you have learned to recognize negative influences on your body profile, you may want to change some things—perhaps aspects of your day-to-day behavior, the way you react to particular situations, how you move, or the way you hold yourself. There are many practical things you can do to bring about change, but bear in mind that this will require patience; transitions in the way we move or think are a reeducation process and do not happen overnight.

Simply being aware of your posture, paying attention to it, and thinking about how you use your body is a big step in the direction of change. This process should help you to recognize personality traits and the areas of your body where tension is being held. Giving some thought to why this tension is present may also help you to resolve deep-seated problems and find your way to a happier and more confident self.

Learning to relax

Being able to relax is essential for reducing stress levels and can go a long way toward preventing the buildup of stress and negative feelings, making you better able to cope with the challenges of daily life. Part of the relaxation process is controlling your breathing. To practice, sit or lie down comfortably in a warm room and breathe slowly and deeply from the abdomen. Feel your chest expand to its maximum capacity and hold your breath briefly before slowly releasing it again. Keep breathing deeply until you feel the tension drain from your body.

CORRECTING YOUR SITTING POSTURE

Many people spend a large part of their lives in a seated position. Sitting puts one-third more pressure on the spine than standing, and poor sitting posture, often encouraged by badly designed chairs, can result in a buildup of tension in the body and lead to back problems. Sitting for prolonged periods leads to muscle fatigue, causing you to slump down farther into your chair as the day progresses. Use the guide below to check and correct your sitting position, and keep reminding yourself of it throughout the day. To reduce muscle fatigue, regularly allow time to stand up and walk around or do a few stretches.

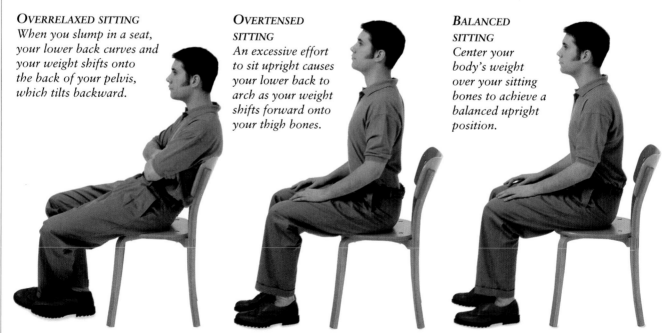

OVERRELAXED SITTING
When you slump in a seat, your lower back curves and your weight shifts onto the back of your pelvis, which tilts backward.

OVERTENSED SITTING
An excessive effort to sit upright causes your lower back to arch as your weight shifts forward onto your thigh bones.

BALANCED SITTING
Center your body's weight over your sitting bones to achieve a balanced upright position.

RELAXING THROUGH VISUALIZATION

This visualization exercise can form part of a tension-releasing regimen. Allow about 15 minutes for the exercise. Picture a scene that you find calming, perhaps a sunny, secluded beach or a tranquil lake. Imagine yourself as an object within that scene, perhaps a piece of driftwood moving lazily with the tide. You are responsive to movement but remain unchanged.

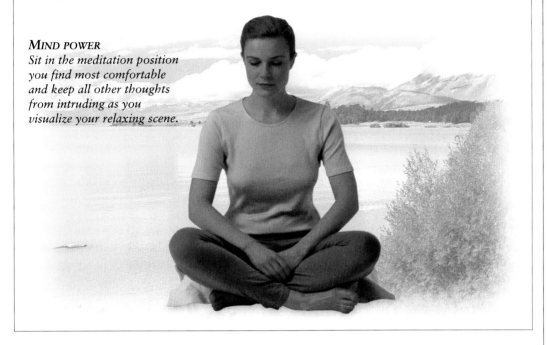

MIND POWER
Sit in the meditation position you find most comfortable and keep all other thoughts from intruding as you visualize your relaxing scene.

The next step is to ease the tension in your muscles. Focus on the muscles of each part of the body in turn, tightening them as you inhale and then slowly relaxing them as you exhale. Start with the muscles in your feet and work up your body, bit by bit, to finish with the face muscles. By the end of this session, all the muscles in your body will feel much more relaxed. Try to set aside at least 15 to 30 minutes each day for a period of total relaxation or meditation.

Changing your posture

Once you feel mentally and physically more relaxed, concentrate on making improvements in your posture. To keep your body in perfect alignment, posture needs to be balanced. Hold your back and neck straight and your head erect as you sit, stand, or walk, so that your upper body weight is carried directly over your spine. When seated, rest your hands in your lap or on the arms of the chair; let them hang easily at your sides as you stand and walk. Keep your movements fluid and your knees, hips, and elbows loose. Roll your feet from your heels to your toes as you walk, trying always to keep your head up, your eyes looking straight ahead, and your body evenly balanced over your legs.

Regular exercise

Long-term stress can lead to entrenched changes in physical shape and posture that will require a program of targeted exercises to undo. Regular physical exercise, such as brisk walking, jogging, dancing, or an active sport, will keep your musculoskeletal system loosened and relaxed and improve circulation to the tissues and joints, thus providing vital nutrients and allowing waste products to flow away easily.

Start each day with a short period of limbering-up exercises, such as jogging in place or a series of easy stretches. This will loosen the joints and increase blood flow to the head, helping to clear your mind of tension in preparation for the day ahead.

At the end of a stressful day, dance to your favorite music or shake out the tension in your body (see right). Follow this activity with a warm, relaxing bath, perhaps adding a few drops each of lavender and rosemary aromatherapy oils to the bathwater.

RELEASING TENSION
Shaking out your muscles is an ideal way to release tension at the end of a stressful day. It can also be used as a wake-up call to your muscles first thing in the morning, as part of a warm-up before exercise, or to release tension in muscles after exercise.

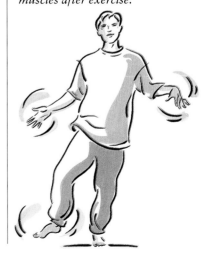

AYURVEDA AND BODY SHAPES

Body reading is an integral part of Ayurveda, an ancient medical system that originated in India and that diagnoses health problems in the context of body type.

Ayurveda, which means the "science of life and longevity" in Sanskrit, is believed to be the oldest medical system in the world and has been practiced in India for more than 5,000 years. It is based on the accumulated knowledge of holy men called *rishis*, or seers of truth, who gained religious and philosophical enlightenment through religious practices and disciplines. This knowledge of life is described in the Vedas, the most ancient of the Hindu holy texts. Many established Eastern systems of philosophy and medicine have been heavily influenced by the principles of Ayurveda. This is why it is sometimes referred to as "the mother of all healing."

Ayurvedic medicine takes a holistic, or whole-body, approach to health, recognizing that many physical symptoms can reflect more wide-ranging and apparently unconnected problems, such as physical misalignments, internal blockages, psychological ailments, and dietary or digestive disorders. Ayurvedic practitioners do not treat symptoms directly but use a combination of therapies, including herbal medicines, massage, diet, and yoga, to correct the imbalances that are causing the underlying disorders.

THE THREE BODY TYPES

In Ayurvedic theory all people are governed by three natural forces, or doshas—*vata,* responsible for movement in the body; *pitta,* which controls digestion and energy; and *kapha,* responsible for the body's structure and stability. The combination of these three forces in all individuals accounts for their metabolism, body shape, and tendency to develop certain kinds of physical disorders. Individuals must know their dominant dosha and keep it balanced with the others.

Typical vata types are thin, with prominent features and cool, dry skin. They are imaginative and highly active people who show flashes of intuition but can be moody. They are prone to nervous disorders, such as anxiety attacks, depression, high blood pressure, stomach upsets, sleeplessness, and cramps.

Pitta types are fair, with a medium build and a ruddy complexion. They tend to be organized, efficient, and warmhearted but can also be short-tempered and intense. Pitta people are prone to skin conditions, such as eczema, sleep disorders, aggressive behavior, hemorrhoids, gallstones, stomach ulcers, and heartburn.

continued on page 44

HEALTH THROUGH KNOWLEDGE

Ayurvedic practitioners believe that only when body, mind, and soul are in harmony is complete health possible. The health system takes account of the human's relationship with the heavens and the cosmos and encompasses science, religion, and philosophy. The name *Ayurveda* literally means "science of life," from *ayu,* meaning "life" and *veda,* meaning "knowledge." In order for us to receive this knowledge, traditionally reserved for the Gods and the enlightened, the three doshas—vata, pitta, and kapha—must be in balance, a state achieved through practicing Ayurveda.

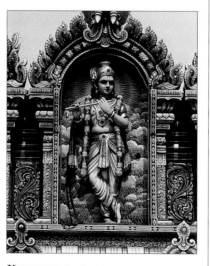

KNOWLEDGE OF THE GODS
Ayurvedic philosophy states that all knowledge comes from the almighty Hindu god, Krishna.

HOW TO DETERMINE YOUR AYURVEDIC BODY TYPE

The following questionnaire can help you to determine which Ayurvedic body type, or types, most closely matches you. Starting with vata, look at each of the characteristics listed and circle the number that you feel is most appropriate for you. Add up the results of the test so that you have a total figure. Do the pitta and kapha tests in the same way until you have a total for each of the three sections, then score your results.

VATA

	RARELY	SOMETIMES	OFTEN
Light build	0	1	2
Quick to act	0	1	2
Poor memory	0	1	2
Slow to decide	0	1	2
Quick to learn	0	1	2
Lively	0	1	2
Enthusiastic	0	1	2
Excitable	0	1	2
Energetic	0	1	2
Receptive to ideas	0	1	2
Talkative	0	1	2
Sensitive to cold	0	1	2
Anxious	0	1	2
Irregular eating and sleeping habits	0	1	2
Changing moods	0	1	2
Total			

PITTA

	RARELY	SOMETIMES	OFTEN
Medium build	0	1	2
Hearty eater	0	1	2
Efficient	0	1	2
Punctilious	0	1	2
Regular habits	0	1	2
Strong-willed	0	1	2
Irritable	0	1	2
Intolerant	0	1	2
Impatient	0	1	2
Blunt speaking	0	1	2
Tenacious	0	1	2
Self-critical	0	1	2
Enjoy a challenge	0	1	2
Dislike warm, humid weather	0	1	2
Sweat easily	0	1	2
Total			

KAPHA

	RARELY	SOMETIMES	OFTEN
Heavy build	0	1	2
Prone to overweight	0	1	2
Abundant, thick dark hair	0	1	2
Smooth, pale skin	0	1	2
Calm and placid	0	1	2
Sound sleeper	0	1	2
Slow to anger	0	1	2
Slow to learn	0	1	2
Good memory	0	1	2
Good with money	0	1	2
Dislike being cold	0	1	2
Gentle	0	1	2
Cheerful	0	1	2
Affectionate	0	1	2
Slow eater	0	1	2
Total			

HOW TO SCORE

To find your dominating dosha, compare your scores for the three tests and see if one outweighs the other two or if two dosha types predominate. Perhaps all three scores are quite close together. Use the following sample results as a guide:

Vata 20, Pitta 18, Kapha 10 = Vata-pitta type

Vata 23, Pitta 10, Kapha 5 = Vata type

Vata 9, Pitta 8, Kapha 7 = Vata-pitta-kapha type

Vata 10, Pitta 8, Kapha 22 = Kapha type

Vata 10, Pitta 17, Kapha 19 = Pitta-kapha type

When you know your dominant dosha type, you will be able to apply Ayurveda more accurately to your lifestyle. However, to understand the full significance of your body type, it is best to seek the advice of an experienced Ayurvedic practitioner, especially if your characteristics are spread across the three types more or less equally.

TEN-DAY PURIFICATION DIET

The first step in practicing Ayurveda is a 10-day purification diet of light, easily digested foods. A practitioner will devise a diet tailored to your dosha, or you can use the diet shown here as part of a self-help program. The diet will improve digestion and allow your body to expel toxins and waste products, known as *ama* in Ayurvedic terms. Listed below are the foods allowed during the diet, plus brief diet guidelines. After 10 days, gradually start to eat normally, following a diet suitable to your dosha type.

▶ *Fruits: orange, banana, mango, and papaya. Oranges should be sucked rather than eaten in segments because this aids salivation and boosts the metabolism.*

▶ *Vegetables: potatoes, carrots, broccoli, cauliflower, beets, and cooked leafy greens.*

▶ *Beans and rice: lentils, mung beans (the latter are high in protein), brown rice.*

▶ *Flavorings: turmeric and ginger.*

▶ *The only bread allowed is chapati made with whole-grain flour.*

▶ *Avoid roasted, fried, fatty, sour, and uncooked foods; fish, pork, and beef; cheese, yogurt, and other milk products; and sweet foods.*

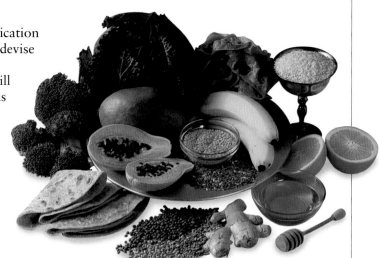

DIET GUIDELINES

On waking and at intervals during the day, drink warm boiled water with a little lemon and honey added. This drink stimulates the metabolism and the elimination of ama. During the diet it is recommended that you skip breakfast unless you are very hungry, in which case you can eat a chapati or drink freshly squeezed fruit juice. Lunch should be the main meal of the day and consist of a light, warm meal, such as rice and vegetables. Skip dinner or have a light meal of fruit juice or a small bowl of soup made with grains or vegetables.

Those who fit the kapha type tend to be heavily built, with thick, wavy hair and pale skin. They are easygoing, compassionate, and affectionate but lack motivation and are prone to allergies, obesity, and heart disease.

Each dosha is situated in particular parts of the body. Vata is based in the large intestine, bones, ears, and thighs; pitta is found in the small intestine, stomach, and blood; and kapha is found in the chest, lungs, and spinal fluid. All three doshas exist in the body in combinations that match the individual's constitution. According to Ayurvedic principles, when the doshas are balanced in accordance with the individual's personality, that person is fit and healthy, but when the doshas are out of balance, physical and mental disorders arise. Ayurvedic medicine aims to restore the doshas to equilibrium.

AYURVEDIC THERAPY

An Ayurvedic doctor will recommend a daily health regimen tailored to your body type and physical condition or disorder. The practitioner may recommend starting with a 10-day purification diet (see box, above), designed to rid the body of waste products and harmful toxins, known as *ama*. This usually includes one or two light meals a day, consisting of rice, cooked vegetables, beans, and soup but no meat, fish, dairy products, or fried or roasted foods.

Foods for dosha types

After this 10-day period, the regular diet is based on the individual's constitution type in order to balance the dominating dosha with the other two. For example, vata types should have stews, pasta, rice, wheat products, and baked dishes but avoid salads, raw vegetables, and most beans. Vata types are prone to digestive problems, so it is important that their meals be easily digestible. People of this type should also eat in a pleasant environment because they are sensitive to stress. Pitta types should eat vegetables, fruits, dairy products, and poultry but avoid all red meat, yogurt, and hot spices. Pitta types tend to overeat and can take the edge off their appetite with bitter and astringent foods or by eating at regular intervals and not skipping meals. Kapha types should eat low-fat spicy dishes, fruits, vegetables, and beans, but should avoid rice, wheat products, and most meats. Cold weather can unbalance kapha types, so hot and spicy foods are recommended in winter.

Whole-body massage

Another aspect of Ayurveda is regular massage with oils to stimulate the elimination of toxins and waste products by increasing the circulation. Massage also relaxes the body and mind and is very effective when used regularly. Vata types should include a daily self-massage in their routine, whereas for pitta and kapha types, two or three times a week is sufficient. Cold-pressed sesame oil is recommended, but pitta types and those with skin problems are advised to use olive, coconut, or sweet almond oil instead. You can find these oils in pharmacies and health food stores.

To improve the oil's suitability for massage and lengthen its storage life, heat it gently for a few minutes in a saucepan to

Pathway to health

Yoga exercises, or *asanas*, are an important part of Ayurvedic practice, helping to unite the body and mind and balance the three doshas. The *asanas* help ease tensed muscles, tone the internal organs, and improve flexibility. If you are completely new to yoga, you will find it very helpful to attend a class; many adult education centers and health clubs run classes for all levels of ability, from beginning to advanced. The teacher will be able to assess your capabilities and advise you on correct execution. As the weeks go by, your flexibility will improve immensely and you will gain enough knowledge to practice the exercises safely at home as part of a daily routine.

about 110°C (230°F). Use a thermometer to check the temperature or add a couple of drops of water to the hot oil; if it sizzles, the temperature is about right. Prepare about 150 ml (5 fl oz) of oil at a time and decant it

---

RULES FOR HEALTHY EATING

In addition to dietary rules, Ayurveda places great store in the way food is eaten.

▶ *Eat at the same time each day, allowing at least three hours between meals.*

▶ *Try to make the midday meal the main one of the day and eat only light meals at other times.*

▶ *Always sit down to eat and avoid distractions, such as the television, so you can concentrate on your food.*

▶ *Eat in a calm, relaxed atmosphere and chew your food slowly and thoroughly.*

▶ *Stop eating as soon as you start to feel satisfied and don't allow yourself to become too full.*

SPORTS FOR EACH DOSHA TYPE

Ayurvedic exercise aims for balance between body and mind and tends to be gentle and enriching without placing undue stress on the body. Walks in the countryside and controlled exercise like yoga are ideal. Ayurvedic exercise can also take the form of a sport but should not be competitive. Furthermore, not all sports are thought to be suitable for all dosha types; it is believed that your physique and personality make you more suited to certain activities than others.

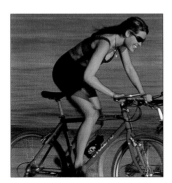

ENERGETIC VATA
Slim and energetic, vata types are best suited to aerobics, cycling, walking, and more graceful forms of dancing, such as ballet.

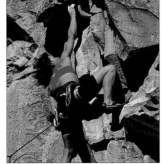

QUICK-WITTED PITTA
Medium-built pitta types do well with jogging, horse back riding, orienteering, swimming, skiing, and mountaineering.

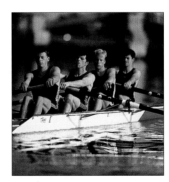

PERSEVERING KAPHA
Kapha types are suited to sports that require control and endurance, such as fencing, football, running, rowing, tennis, and weight lifting.

ALTERNATE NOSTRIL BREATHING

To achieve rhythmic breathing, Ayurveda recommends the yogic practice of alternate nostril breathing, or *pranayama*. Wear loose, comfortable clothing and sit in a cross-legged position on the floor or in a chair, with your back and neck straight but not tense. Close your eyes and breathe deeply a few times, concentrating on the breath in your nostrils. When you are ready, open your eyes and follow steps 1 and 2 below. Continue the sequence for about 5 minutes, then finish by sitting still for a minute, breathing normally.

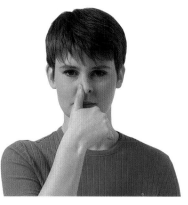

1 *Lightly close the airway of your right nostril with your right thumb. Breathe out slowly through your open left nostril. Breathe in after a few seconds through the left nostril, then pinch the nostril shut.*

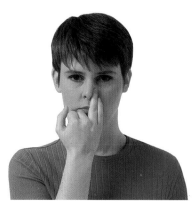

2 *At the same time, release the right nostril and the air you are holding. Breathe out slowly through the right nostril and hold your breath for a few seconds. Breathe in, close the nostril shut again, and repeat the process.*

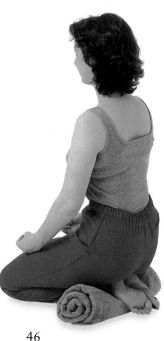

*EASY MEDITATION POSE
This yoga pose is an ideal position for breathing and meditation exercises. Kneel with your feet straight and your sitting bones resting evenly on your heels. Placing a rolled blanket under your feet and/or a cushion over your heels may improve comfort and enable you to maintain the position longer.*

into an airtight jar for future use. The oil is applied all over the body before the massage begins, so that it has time to be absorbed by the skin. The body is then massaged from head to foot using gentle, circular movements of the hands.

Yoga exercise

Regular yoga exercises (see page 138) are an important element of Ayurvedic therapy. Yoga enhances suppleness and mobility, relieves muscle tension, and can alleviate such problems as migraines and other headaches, back pain, stiff joints, and circulatory disorders. A yoga session usually begins with stretching and bending to prepare the body; these are followed by assuming and holding special body positions, or *asanas*. Regular, even, and deep breathing is an important part of yoga.

Breathing and meditation

Ayurveda stresses the importance of proper breathing. The alternate nostril breathing exercise (see box, above) called *pranayama*, is designed to control and enhance the flow of natural energy, or *prana*, in the body,

leading to good health. Practiced for five minutes each morning and evening, the exercise prepares the body for the final stage of the Ayurvedic regimen—meditation.

Just as physical waste products can build up in the body, so too can emotional wastes accumulate. Meditation is the process by which the body rids itself of this emotional product. A daily meditation session lasting 15 minutes is usually sufficient, although it can be longer. Choose a comfortable position, such as the one shown far left, or sit upright in a chair with your back straight. Rest your hands on your thighs or in your lap. It may help to have an object nearby—a candle, for example—that you can focus on at first. Breathe calmly as you look at the candle and then close your eyes and hold the image in your head, letting your thoughts drift. Don't try to control your thoughts or stop other thoughts from intruding, but don't dwell on anything either. As your thoughts become more unfocused, breathe more deeply. To end the session, rest quietly for a few moments with your eyes open while you evaluate any changes you have experienced in yourself.

BODY-READING THERAPIES

Body-reading therapies aim to identify and correct the poor posture and restricted movement that can cause some physical disorders, as well as mental and emotional problems.

Most therapies take account of the physical symptoms of a disorder in order to arrive at a diagnosis. But certain forms of therapy, sometimes known as body-reading therapies, also put great store on close study of the patient's posture in order to discover an underlying cause of the physical condition.

Body-reading therapies are based on the belief that there is a close connection between a patient's emotional and psychological problems and his or her stance and movement patterns. By correcting any faults in the person's posture and way of moving—the physical manifestations of the problem—the therapist aims to alleviate the underlying problem itself. The Alexander technique and Rolfing are two of the most widely practiced body-reading therapies. Similar techniques, such as Hellerwork, LooyenWork, and Watsu, are also gaining in popularity.

ALEXANDER TECHNIQUE

One of the first people to recognize the connection between inner psychological states and outward physical problems was not a therapist at all but an Australian actor, F. Matthias Alexander. Alexander began to lose his voice on stage and yet not at other

---

ALEXANDER TECHNIQUE APPLIED TO SWIMMING

The Alexander technique can highlight ways to improve posture and movement during activities to prevent the buildup of tension. The most common fault in swimming is to swim with your head out of the water, which puts pressure on the spine. Taking lessons and practicing can help you to overcome this problem and to establish a breathing pattern that will also improve your swimming technique.

▶ *Invest in some good-quality goggles to protect your eyes from chlorine or salt in the water. Practice with them in shallow water where you can stand up if necessary.*

▶ *To avoid gasping when you lift your head out of the water to inhale, exhale while your face is in the water, releasing the air from your mouth very slowly.*

▶ *Gradually increase the number of strokes you do with your face in the water. In the front crawl, do four or five strokes, then lift your head to the side for a breath.*

▶ *By swimming with your head level with your body, you will maintain correct body alignment and achieve better forward propulsion.*

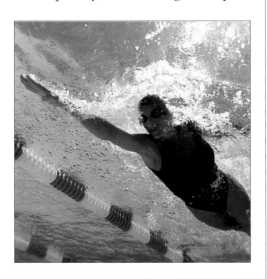

FINDING A PRACTITIONER

Alternative therapies are becoming more and more popular as the number of success stories grows. However, it is advisable to do some research before signing up for a course of treatments.

▶ *Ask friends, family, and health professionals for recommendations.*

▶ *Find out what the initials after a name stand for, if they are qualifications, and whether they were earned at an accredited establishment.*

▶ *Find out if there is a governing body for the therapy of your choice. This organization may provide a list of registered therapists in your area.*

▶ *Call the practitioner and find out as much as possible about the therapy, including any contraindications. Trust your instincts; if you don't like the therapist's manner or find him or her vague, you will be less likely to benefit from the treatment.*

times, and so he studied himself while rehearsing in front of a mirror to see if he could discover the cause of the problem. He noticed that the stress of acting caused him to shrink down into himself and lower his head, which constricted his neck and throat and obstructed his breathing. By constantly observing himself and consciously correcting the postural faults he detected, he was able to reduce his feelings of stress, restore his normal voice, and develop a healthier, more natural posture.

Alexander developed his observations into a comprehensive therapy—the Alexander technique—which became very popular, particularly among actors and orators, and is now widely practiced in Europe and America. The technique aims to improve posture and mobility and promote physical and mental harmony. It is most often used to relieve anxiety and stress and to alleviate back and neck pain, but can also be used to treat headaches, heart disease, respiratory conditions, intestinal disorders such as irritable bowel syndrome, and arthritis.

Before starting treatment, a teacher of Alexander technique will study the way the patient sits, stands, and walks. The teacher will be looking for postural errors, such as slouching or rounded shoulders, arched or stiff back, or the head held too far back.

While the student is seated or standing, the teacher will then very gently manipulate the body into the correct alignment and give advice on healthy posture. The teacher will also explain how to recognize and relieve stress. For lasting physical benefits it is important that the subject put the teacher's advice into practice every day and not just in the treatment room.

ROLFING

Rolfing massage and manipulation techniques are used to improve posture and alleviate deep-seated tension, chronic muscle and joint problems, and other physical ailments. The method is sometimes called deep-tissue bodywork because the therapist manipulates the deep muscular and connective tissues, as well as the surface tissues, of the body. In particular, Rolfing concentrates on a form of connective tissue called fascia, which surrounds and binds the muscle fibers and links muscles and bones (see pages 20–21).

An American biochemist, Dr. Ida Rolf (1896–1979), developed Rolfing. She discovered that fascia adapts to your posture and movement patterns and can become fixed, locking you into bad postural habits. For example, if you habitually hunch your shoulders, the fascia will tighten into this position, making it difficult to break the habit. Dr. Rolf believed that to improve posture, the fascia has to be stretched and manipulated into the correct positions, using various Rolfing techniques, so that the connective tissue adapts to the change and supports you in the new healthy posture.

Many postural problems in which the body is out of alignment are believed to be caused by deep-seated emotional traumas. For example, feeling depressed could cause you to adopt a round-shouldered and compacted stance. Dr. Rolf believed that by correcting these postural problems, she could also release the emotional traumas that caused them in the first place.

A Rolfer will study the way a patient sits, stands, and walks around to diagnose misalignments that need to be corrected. The practitioner will also take a photograph of

AREAS OF
MISALIGNMENT
Body-reading therapies, including Rolfing, the Alexander technique, and osteopathy, start with a complete posture assessment. The practitioner looks at the alignment of your body while you are standing, sitting, and walking.

The drawing at right shows some common areas of misalignment. The person's weight is shifted onto the left side, putting stress on the weight-bearing joints of the knee and ankle. In an effort to compensate, the spine has become curved and the ribs on the left side cramped, thus restricting breathing.

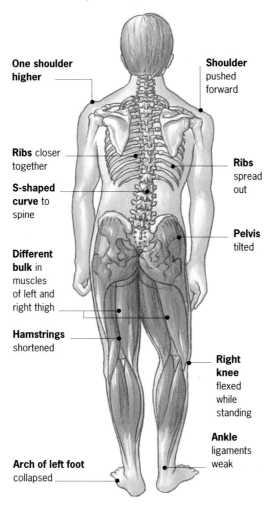

One shoulder higher

Ribs closer together

S-shaped curve to spine

Different bulk in muscles of left and right thigh

Hamstrings shortened

Arch of left foot collapsed

Shoulder pushed forward

Ribs spread out

Pelvis tilted

Right knee flexed while standing

Ankle ligaments weak

An Unassertive Secretary

Unassertive people are often taken for granted. They may be given tasks that others prefer to avoid and may be passed over for promotion in favor of less able but more assertive people. The resulting frustration can manifest itself in physical ailments, such as chronic muscle pain and headaches. Treating the symptoms alone is not sufficient; a fundamental change in attitude is required.

Jan is a 45-year-old secretary at a pharmaceutical company who has worked for her current boss for more than 11 years. Jan is regarded as a conscientious worker by her colleagues; she is prepared to put in long hours without complaint and often takes on extra unpaid tasks, such as organizing company social events. Despite her good reputation within the company, she has never been offered a promotion to a more senior level and has seen other, less experienced people promoted above her. Her lack of progress has left her increasingly despondent, and she has started suffering from regular headaches and pain in her shoulders. Recently the pain has prevented her from playing in her regular weekly tennis match.

WHAT SHOULD JAN DO?

Jan's aches and pains are possibly stress-related and linked to feelings of low self-esteem. Because of her lack of assertiveness, co-workers take her for granted. Unless she can increase her assertiveness, this situation is unlikely to change. Besides taking better care of her own needs, Jan needs to redress the imbalance of work and relaxation in her life, making more time for her interests and to take care of her health. Reintroducing regular exercise into her life could help her manage pain better. A friend suggested that Hellerwork might help because the therapy is designed to deal with underlying emotional and psychological problems as well as physical disorders.

Action Plan

WORK
Attend an assertiveness course to learn how to confront colleagues and managers positively about areas of dissatisfaction.

EMOTIONAL HEALTH
Accept that unexpressed emotions need to be released somehow. Learn how to use assertion to express feelings in a positive way.

FITNESS
Allocate time each day to some form of exercise, such as yoga, that will relieve tension and stretch muscles.

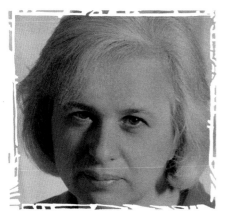

FITNESS
Neglecting to exercise regularly can exacerbate muscle tension.

WORK
Being unassertive at work can lead to missed promotions and a lack of recognition, in the long term causing frustration and anger.

EMOTIONAL HEALTH
Repressed emotions can cause tension in the body, which can lead to misaligned posture and painful muscle problems.

HOW THINGS TURNED OUT FOR JAN

Jan saw a Hellerworker, whose analysis revealed long-held anger and frustration. He used massage and manipulation to ease the muscle tension and talked to Jan about the need to release her pent-up feelings. He also assigned daily exercises. After the first session Jan felt very emotional, and she thought hard about areas of dissatisfaction in her life. By the end of treatment, her pain had lessened, and she had resolved to take an assertiveness course.

Origins

Hellerwork is the brainchild of former aerospace engineer Joseph Heller. It is based closely on Rolfing, the body-work system founded in the mid-1960s by Dr. Ida Rolf (see page 48). Heller studied under Dr. Rolf and became the first president of the Rolf Institute in 1975, leaving to set up his own system of bodywork therapy in 1978. This combines tissue manipulation with posture and movement education and also places considerable emphasis on understanding the memories and emotional attitudes that surface during therapy.

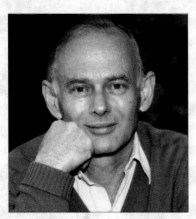

JOSEPH HELLER (B. 1940)
Heller studied several different healing therapies, including Rolfing, Structural Patterning, and bioenergetics, before devising his unique form of bodywork.

the patient before treatment begins to highlight the problem areas, such as stooped shoulders or arched back, and then another picture after the course of treatment has been completed to show the changes that Rolfing has brought about.

In addition to improved posture and relief from physical problems, such as neck and back pain, patients who have undergone a course of treatment often report increased energy and vitality.

HELLERWORK

Hellerwork is a form of deep-tissue body therapy, similar in some respects to Rolfing, based on the idea of the body, mind, and spirit being inseparable. It aims to help a person attain an optimal state of well-being. Hellerwork is helpful for relieving chronic tension and such nerve disorders as fibromyalgia and repetitive stress syndrome, but it concentrates also on helping a patient to move more naturally and to deal with underlying emotional problems. A Hellerwork therapist questions a patient throughout treatment to try to uncover any traumas or conflicts. Hellerwork is thought to be particularly successful in treating people suffering from severe emotional trauma—for example, individuals who have been involved in an accident or disaster or have been the victim of a violent crime.

LOOYENWORK

The theory that psychological trauma is stored in the physical body is explored to an even greater degree in LooyenWork. This body-reading therapy was founded by Ted Looyen, a psychotherapist who failed to find relief for his own chronic back pain in massage and other manipulation therapies.

LooyenWork includes physical manipulation, but it is directed more toward relieving chronic emotional tension and resolving psychological conflicts, such as those arising from divorce or parental rejection. To uncover these deep-seated traumas, the therapist reads the way the subject sits and stands and how his or her muscles move.

Patients are counseled on the emotional changes they are undergoing while the therapist manipulates the body to alleviate the outward physical signs of emotional tension. In addition, therapists aim to enhance the patient's confidence, self-esteem, and ability to concentrate.

WATSU

Watsu is a form of water therapy based on the Eastern massage technique known as shiatsu. In shiatsu the therapist uses fingers, thumbs, hands, arms, elbows, and even the knees and feet to free blockages in the flow of energy through the body's energy pathways. In Watsu a similar form of massage and manipulation is carried out while the subject floats in a warm pool. Being immersed in warm water takes the pressure off the patient's musculoskeletal system, particularly the spine and joints, making it easier for the therapist to stretch and realign the muscles and connective tissue.

Watsu aims to release stress and ease muscle tension and physical aches and pains and to heal the spirit, mind, and body as well. It was devised by Harold Dull, an American poet who believed it would be beneficial to unite the healing arts of shiatsu and acupressure with the therapeutic effects of warm water. The combination of manipulation, massage, and water therapy is said to strengthen blood circulation, the lymphatic system, and the immune response, and to ease digestive and breathing problems. It is believed to help relieve psychological problems, such as stress, insomnia, anxiety, and even addictions. It has also been used to improve the mobility of physically and mentally disabled people.

CHAPTER 3

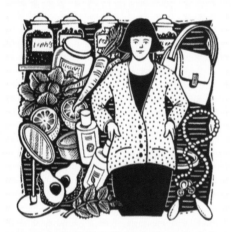

LIFESTYLE AND YOUR SHAPE

*Making sure your body is fueled for
exercise through a well-balanced diet will
improve your health and help you to reach your
shaping-up goals. In the meantime, there is a lot
you can do to enhance your appearance by taking
care of your skin and focusing on clothes that
work with your shape, not against it.*

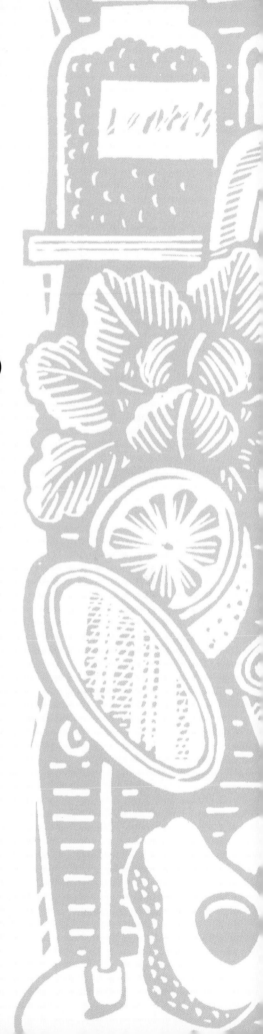

HEALTHY EATING FOR A BETTER SHAPE

A well-balanced diet is the starting point of any shaping-up regimen. It should provide the fuel you need for exercise and all the nutrients your body requires to maintain good health.

People are often surprised to discover after starting a regular exercise program that they have a greater appetite than before. A diet for exercise should not leave you feeling deprived or hungry, but it is important to bring some discipline and planning into your eating routine. It can be tempting and all too easy to increase fat intake, but it is healthier to eat low-fat foods, in particular those that are high in carbohydrates, which will give you energy for increased physical activity.

It is not just a question of what foods you choose but also when you eat them. You should eat at regular intervals throughout the day and avoid skipping meals. Snacks are fine as long as they are low in saturated fat and sugar. Fruit, whole-grain crackers, and low-fat yogurt are good choices.

One approach to planning an exercise diet is to divide food into five main groups—starchy grain foods, such as pasta, bread, cereal, and rice; fruits and vegetables; high-protein foods, including meat, fish, poultry, eggs, and legumes; low-fat dairy products; and fatty and sugary foods (see chart, below left). By eating the right amount of food from each group to meet your energy needs, you will also ensure that your body receives all the essential nutrients it requires.

Aim to eat more fruits, vegetables, and whole grains while reducing your consumption of high-fat and high-sugar foods. Overall calorie requirements vary from one person to another, depending on basic metabolic rate and amount of activity. A young active adult will need a higher calorie intake than an equally active older person, for example.

THE RIGHT BALANCE
This pie chart represents the right proportions of the main food groups in a balanced diet. Fruits and vegetables should make up about one-third, while grains should make up another third. Dairy foods should represent up to one-sixth, and meat, fish, legumes, and eggs should equal about another sixth. This leaves little room for high-fat and sugary foods, which should be kept to a minimum.

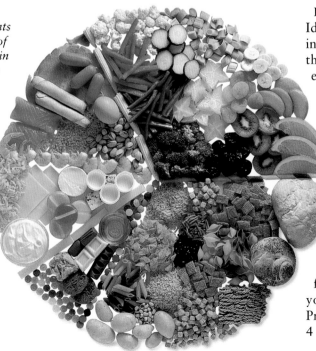

FOODS FOR WEIGHT GAIN AND LOSS
Ideally, weight gain should result from increased muscle rather than fat. To achieve this, you must combine a well-balanced exercise regimen with a nutritious diet that provides more energy than your body burns. Mealtimes should be at regular intervals, and you should never skip any. If you can, try to eat bigger portions at each meal, but if this is difficult, you can intersperse meals with healthy snacks at midmorning, mid afternoon, and midevening.

The only way to lose weight is to consume fewer calories than your body needs for normal bodily processes and physical activity. The fuel your body uses for energy comes from calories in the food you eat and from fat stored in the body. Protein and carbohydrate in food both yield 4 calories per gram, whereas fat contains

9 calories per gram. A few foods—butter, margarine, and vegetable oils, for instance—are mostly fat; some, such as fruit and pasta, contain largely carbohydrate; and egg whites are almost pure protein. Most foods, however, are a mixture of all three components in varying proportions. Because fat contains more than twice the calories per gram than carbohydrate and protein, it makes sense to cut back on fatty foods and go for the less calorie-dense carbohydrates and protein in order to lose weight.

Alcohol is also fairly high in calories—about 7 calories per gram. But these calories are empty ones; that is, they provide no nutrients, and they contribute readily to fat storage in the body.

FOODS FOR EXERCISE

To sustain peak performance during exercise, you need an adequate amount of carbohydrate—in the form of glucose and glycogen—stored in your body. The body will first burn the glucose circulating in the blood, then the glycogen stored in muscles and the liver. After 20 minutes or so of steady aerobic exercise, the body starts to burn fat stores as well.

To maintain an adequate supply of glucose for moderate to vigorous exercise, most people need to obtain 55 to 65 percent of their calories from foods high in carbohydrates, especially the starches in grain foods like rice, bread, and pasta.

Gaining muscle calls for foods that are high in complete protein, such as fish, meat, poultry, eggs, or vegetarian equivalents of animal protein; examples of the last are soy products and other kinds of legumes combined with grains. Low-fat milk and dairy foods are good sources as well. (You also must do regular resistance exercise to build muscle.) Contrary to what some people believe, however, you don't need large quantities of dietary protein to build muscle mass and maintain strength. Only 10 to 12 percent of daily calories needs to come from protein, which for an adult who weighs 140 pounds is about 50 grams.

An intake of excess protein has several drawbacks. It increases the excretion of calcium and other minerals from the body and puts extra strain on the liver and kidneys, which have to process unused protein. Any remaining unused protein is stored as fat.

continued on page 56

THE IMPORTANCE OF CALCIUM

Calcium is essential for healthy bones. Most bones begin in the embryo as cartilage and are gradually replaced by hard bone. This process, known as ossification, starts when the fetus is about 7 weeks old and continues throughout childhood and into adulthood, with maximum bone mass achieved by about age 30. From about age 35 on, bone density gradually decreases, and in old age, thinning can lead to osteoporosis (see page 25). Both women and men are advised to increase their calcium intake after age 65 because an increased loss of bone density is common at this time.

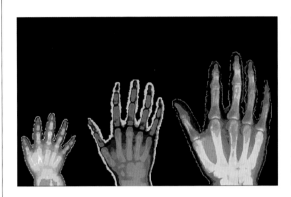

BONE GROWTH
These hand X-rays, at 30 months (left), 6 years (middle) and 19 years (right) show the hardening of bone in progress. Notice how the spaces between bones lessen as more cartilage ossifies.

CALCIUM CONTENT OF SOME FOODS

The newest recommendations for calcium are 1,000 mg per day for most adults, 1,500 mg after age 65. It is best to obtain it from the diet, but supplements may be needed.

TYPE OF FOOD	MG PER 100 G	MG PER TYPICAL SERVING
DAIRY PRODUCTS		
Milk (skim)	120	300 mg per 8-ounce serving
Cheese (Cheddar)	728	400 mg per 2-ounce serving
Yogurt (low-fat)	182	430 mg per 8-ounce serving
LEGUMES AND NUTS		
Soybeans (fresh)	145	130 mg per ½-cup serving
Chickpeas (dried)	48	40 mg per ½-cup serving
Almonds (dry-roasted)	360	100 mg per 1-ounce serving
VEGETABLES & FRUITS		
Green beans	46	52 mg per 4-ounce serving
Kale	72	84 mg per 4-ounce serving
Broccoli	48	65 mg per 5-ounce serving
Apricots (dried)	67	58 mg per 3-ounce serving
Orange	40	56 mg per medium-size fruit
FISH		
Salmon (canned with bones)	213	180 mg per 3-ounce serving
Sardines (canned with bones)	378	215 mg per 2-ounce serving
Tuna (fresh albacore)	31	43 mg per 5-ounce serving

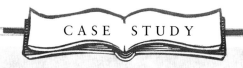

CASE STUDY

A Fatigued Mother

It is possible to get the balance of exercise and diet wrong, particularly when the main reason for working out is to lose weight. Snacking with the wrong foods or at the wrong times and not refueling after a workout, perhaps because your appetite is suppressed by exercise, can lead to fatigue and often little in the way of weight loss.

Anna, 33 years old, is married to Roger, an advertising executive, and they have two children. Thomas is 5 and very boisterous and seems to manage on very little sleep. Laura is 3 years old and has become very clingy since starting nursery school. Roger's pressured work life means that the care of the children falls almost solely on Anna's shoulders.

Anna has recently joined a gym, determined to lose weight before her birthday in two months' time. She decided that a combination of workouts and strict dieting would be the answer. The easiest time for her to

exercise is while Laura is at nursery school, but Anna often arrives at the gym already exhausted. Her workout, devised by the gym instructor, starts with with a warmup, followed by 40 minutes of aerobic work on machines, then 20 minutes using weights, and ends with a cooldown.

Anna tries to have breakfast cereal with the children but often manages nothing more than a cup of coffee. While Laura has her lunch, Anna grabs a sandwich or eats leftovers from the refrigerator. She spends the afternoon playing with Laura before picking up Thomas. The children

have an early supper, and Anna, who is starving by now, picks at what they are having and finishes off what they leave. (She doesn't think this amounts to much in the way of calories.) The next few hours are chaotic as Anna prepares supper for Roger and herself and gets the children ready for bed. When Roger gets home, supper is ready but Anna is too exhausted to eat much.

What really puzzles Anna is that for all her activity, her weight is not going down very much. She is very tempted to quit the gym; at least then, she feels, she won't be so tired.

FAMILY
Young children can be very demanding on their parents' time, and this can be particularly wearing when one parent is providing the bulk of the care.

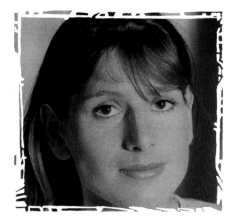

HEALTH
Your body should receive all the vitamins and minerals it needs from a healthy, balanced diet. Constant fatigue may be a sign of a health problem and should be checked out by a doctor.

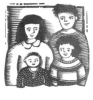
DIET
It is easy to neglect your diet when you have a hectic lifestyle. Snacking can easily lead to a high fat and sugar intake and a lack of essential nutrients, such as calcium and iron.

EXERCISE
Weight loss can be achieved gradually by combining exercise with a sensible weight-loss diet. Overdoing the exercise can be counterproductive and lead to fatigue.

STRESS
Setting unrealistic goals can lead to increased levels of stress and subsequent irritability. Children react to this, raising stress levels further.

WHAT SHOULD ANNA DO?

Anna has set herself unrealistic targets, both in her weight loss and her exercise program. To achieve a shaping-up goal and retain it, changes in diet and exercise need to be permanent and take into consideration existing pressures, such as work and family. Anna needs to discuss her situation and requirements with the gym instructor so they can devise a more suitable exercise plan in terms of how often and how hard she works out.

Anna's diet is very haphazard and probably contains more calories than she realizes but not enough nutrients. By eating little or nothing at breakfast, Anna is not fueling her body for exercise. Similarly, by not eating a well-balanced meal after exercise, she is missing out on the best time to refuel her body. With such irregular eating habits, she is also more likely to reach for unhealthy snacks.

It could be that Anna's fatigue is due in part to insufficient iron in her diet. Iron deficiency anemia is common in women of childbearing age. Anna should see her doctor for a blood test to check out this possibility. At the same time she should have her weight checked and seek advice about how much weight she actually needs to lose. Many women strive for a body weight that is below what is normally recommended for their height.

Action Plan

FAMILY
Talk to the nursery school teacher about Laura's clinginess. Ask Roger to help out some with the children; perhaps he could look after them first thing in the morning or do the bedtime routine on weekends.

DIET
Record in a diary all food and beverages consumed each day to see how much is actually being eaten. Make an effort to eat breakfast every morning and increase carbohydrate intake at lunchtime. Refuel with some carbohydrate, such as fruit juice, right after exercise.

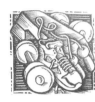

EXERCISE
Speak to the gym instructor about changing the program to a less intense one for the time being. Reduce the number of gym sessions to a more manageable level.

STRESS
Assess whether weight loss is actually necessary by calculating BMI, and draw up a workable weight-control plan. Make time during the day to relax.

HEALTH
Make an appointment to see the doctor to discuss constant fatigue and possibility of anemia. Also ask for advice on diet improvements (perhaps seek a referral to a dietitian) and a recommendation on ideal weight for height.

HOW THINGS TURNED OUT FOR ANNA

Anna talked to her gym instructor, who reduced the intensity of her program. Because the rest of her life was very active, he decided she would get sufficient benefit from working out twice a week.

She also went to see her doctor, who told her that she was not anemic but her blood hemoglobin level could be better. He gave her a list of iron-rich foods and recommended including more of them in her diet. The doctor also told Anna sternly never to skip breakfast and suggested that she was exaggerating her weight problem; her plan to lose 15 pounds would actually make her a little underweight.

Anna followed her new exercise program faithfully and found it more enjoyable. She also realized after reading her food diary why she hadn't lost any weight. Her eating habits are now much better, and she feels that her increased energy levels are due in part to her new eating pattern. She never misses breakfast and eats a well-planned lunch to sustain her energy during the day.

Roger was not aware of how demanding the children had become; together they drew up a plan to allow Anna some time off. As a result, Anna's fatigue is greatly reduced and she is now enjoying life much more. Laura is back to her old sociable self too.

Calories and kilocalories

The energy in food is measured in a unit called a calorie, which is the amount of energy needed to raise the temperature of 1 milliliter of water by 1°C. To overcome the problem of counting in such small units, nutrition and health professionals in the past used the term *kilocalorie* or *Calorie* (with a capital *C*), which equals 1,000 calories. Today, however, it is more common to see the word *calorie* (with a small *c*) indicating this larger unit of measurement.

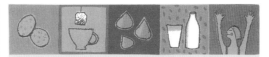

SUPER SHAPER

Chestnuts are an ideal component of a diet geared toward exercise because they are high in energy and low in calories. They have about four times the carbohydrate content of other nuts but only 5 to 10 percent of the fat. They are also good sources of vitamins B_6, C, and folic acid and the minerals potassium, iron, manganese, and magnesium. Chestnuts can be eaten raw but have a slightly bitter flavor. They taste sweeter when roasted, baked, or boiled. They are delicious when served with green vegetables, such as brussels sprouts, and can be pureed for a stuffing or ground up and added to cakes and other sweets.

People who exercise on a regular basis need more protein than those who do not exercise, but this increased requirement is easily met by a normal diet, and there is no need to take a protein supplement.

HEALTHY BONES

During childhood and youth bones become stronger by accumulating calcium (see page 53). This process continues until around age 30, when peak bone mass is reached. After this time a slow decline in bone mass occurs in both men and women as more calcium is lost than is gained through the diet.

The calcium loss accelerates in women after menopause, when the level of estrogen, which helps to maintain bone mass, drops dramatically. Reduced bone mass can lead to osteoporosis, a brittle-bone condition that causes stooped posture, reduced height, and increased risk of bone fractures. The condition, thought to be due in part to genetic factors, currently affects 1 in 4 postmenopausal women and 1 in 12 older men. The incidence of osteoporosis is rising, but there is strong evidence that the rate of bone loss can be reduced by diet and exercise.

To maximize peak bone mass and slow the rate of bone loss, it is important that you exercise regularly throughout life, consume adequate amounts of vitamin D, and maintain a good intake of calcium.

SPACING YOUR MEALS

It is a good idea to make a general plan for your overall food intake each day and then divide it in whatever way works for you. Some experts recommend eating smaller meals and having snacks at regular intervals instead of eating three large meals; by eating more often, you stabilize blood glucose and insulin levels, better control blood cholesterol, and reduce the risk of storing excess fat. Also, each time you eat, you increase your metabolic rate (the energy needed just to keep your body functioning) because of the extra demands of digesting, absorbing, transporting, and metabolizing the food. This can help you maintain your energy balance. Also, spacing your meals and snacks so that you eat soon after exercise will speed recovery by helping to replace the stores of glycogen that have been used during the session.

WHAT TO EAT BEFORE, DURING, AND AFTER AN EXERCISE SESSION

Pre-exercise carbohydrate is useful for persons who work their bodies hard, especially athletes in training. It helps to maintain higher blood sugar levels and delay fatigue. It can also improve endurance, allowing you to train harder for a longer period. A banana, dried fruit, or a sports drink consumed 5 to 30 minutes before training is beneficial if a long, hard session is in store.

Consuming carbohydrate during an exercise session may help increase muscle strength and delay fatigue. Carbohydrate, taken either as a food or a beverage, must be ingested early in a session if you are to reap any benefits. A fruit beverage or sports drink (see opposite page) is the best choice during exercise, and it has a twofold benefit because the fluid also helps prevent dehydration. If you prefer to eat, choose a food recommended for pre-exercise fueling.

The body needs carbohydrate soon after exercise because its store of glycogen is replenished most efficiently in the first one

DID YOU KNOW?

Even in the leanest of athletes there is never a shortage of fat available for fuel. For example, a 154-pound male athlete with a body fat of just 10 percent has a fat store equivalent to 60,000 calories.

to two hours after a training session. If you don't refuel properly, you may feel tired the following day and sluggish during your next exercise session because your muscles have not fully refilled their glycogen stores.

Appetite is often suppressed right after exercise, but most people feel thirsty; fruit juice or a sports drink is a good choice. You can also eat something light, such as a banana or cereal bar, followed two to four hours later by a high-carbohydrate meal.

WATER

Getting enough water is just as important to good health as eating right. Even mild dehydration can interfere with the body's proper functioning, leading to mental and physical sluggishness, headache, poor digestion, loss of appetite, and dizziness. A basic rule of thumb is to drink at least eight glasses of water a day, but some health experts consider this the minimum and suggest that many individuals need more, depending on the weather, their level of activity, where they live (people at high elevations require more

liquid), and how much caffeine and alcohol they consume. During hot weather the body needs more water to keep its temperature regulated. And both caffeine and alcohol are dehydrating; an extra glass of water is needed whenever either is consumed.

Specially formulated sports drinks are becoming increasingly popular, but to be effective the right one must be chosen for each particular need. Research shows that isotonic and hypotonic drinks, which contain 2 to 8 percent carbohydrate plus some sodium, are absorbed faster than water alone and can help prevent dehydration before, during, and after an exercise session. The carbohydrate in the drink will also top up fuel reserves to prevent depletion of glycogen stores, a principal cause of fatigue.

Hypertonic drinks have a higher carbohydrate content (over 10 percent) but are not as effective at rehydrating because the fluid takes longer to enter the bloodstream. Such drinks should be used for refueling after an exercise session or when rehydration is not the top priority.

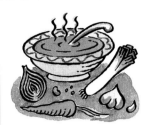

SOUP YOURSELF UP
If you make a variety of warming soups and freeze them, you can have a high-carbohydrate, nutritious meal in a flash. Ideal ingredients include lentils, barley, split peas, and a variety of vegetables.

STOCKING FOODS FOR POWER SNACKS

High-energy snacks and meals can be useful for topping up energy levels a couple of hours before an exercise session or an hour or two after exercise, when the body's refueling is at its most efficient. The aim is to eat or drink foods that are high in carbohydrates, which can be rapidly digested and absorbed by the

body, but low in fat. Make a list of all the foods you like that you can use to make a nutritious high-carbohydrate meal quickly, and keep your kitchen stocked with these food items. Perishables will need replacing each time you go shopping; check your cupboards to see if you are low on any other items.

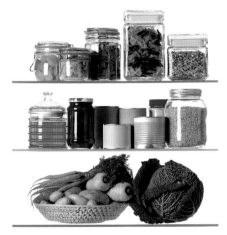

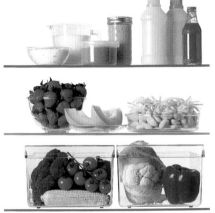

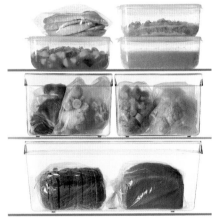

In the Cupboard
Stock breakfast cereals, dried pasta, rice, potatoes, onions, potatoes, dried fruits, peanut butter, honey, and canned tomatoes, beans, fish (in brine or water), pasta sauces, and soups.

In the Refrigerator
Keep on hand low-fat yogurt, low-fat cheese, milk (skim or low-fat), fruit juice, fresh soup and pasta, and fresh fruits and vegetables, such as melon, strawberries, sprouts, and peppers.

In the Freezer
Store bread, rolls, pizza dough, chicken or turkey breasts, fish steaks, frozen vegetables, such as carrots, peas, and cauliflower, and prepared dishes, like casseroles and soups.

SUPPLEMENTS—DO THEY WORK?

There is no shortage of supplements available to the exercising public, but the verdict is still out as to whether some of these dietary aids have any benefits for a shaping-up regimen.

A number of dietary supplements are promoted for enhancing exercise performance, increasing muscle size and strength, reducing fat, and aiding general health. Some are targeted primarily at serious athletes, but other people may be tempted to use them as part of a general diet and exercise program. A few supplements can be beneficial in certain cases, but others have little proven effect and may even be harmful.

MUSCLE-BUILDING PRODUCTS

Many people try supplements that they hope will boost their muscle strength or size, but most of these products are unproven. The best approach to muscle building is a well-balanced diet plus resistance exercise.

Protein supplements

While it is true that protein builds muscle, any that the body doesn't use for normal growth and repair is burned for energy or stored as fat. Except for people who have certain digestive problems, are recovering from an injury, or have very inadequate diets, protein supplements provide little benefit and could be harmful. The toxic waste products from the breakdown of protein are eliminated by the kidneys, and this process can lead to dehydration because more water is needed to get rid of any excess. With healthy kidneys and a good fluid intake, harmful effects are minimized, but the kidneys definitely have to work harder to get rid of excess protein. A high-protein intake can also cause an increased excretion of calcium and other minerals from the body

High-protein diets that include a lot of meat are high in saturated fat as well, which can increase the risk of heart disease. And when the amount of protein in the diet is higher and that of carbohydrate is lower than optimal, the result may be a state of chronic fatigue. This will limit the amount of exercise that can be performed, so even less dietary protein will be converted to muscle.

Body-building chemicals

The male hormones known as androgens belong to a chemical group called steroids, which have a ring-shaped, or steroid, atomic structure. Androgens—testosterone, in particular—have a variety of effects, but they are mainly responsible for the development of male sexual traits at puberty, and they play a part in sexual libido as well.

Androgens are also "anabolic" hormones, which stimulate muscle growth and development. Synthetic drugs called anabolic steroids produce an effect similar to that of androgens, but they have many undesirable physical and psychological side effects that can damage health and may even be life threatening. These include acne, hair loss, oily skin, deepening of the voice, abnormal hair growth on the face and body, masculinization in women, breast enlargement in males, and reduced sperm production. They can also cause personality changes, liver damage, and heart disease. Anabolic steroids should not be confused, however, with corticosteroid drugs, also known as steroids, which are used to treat inflammatory conditions, such as rheumatoid arthritis, and other disorders.

Claims that certain supplements made principally from plant extracts boost the body's production of testosterone and thus increase muscle mass, are unsupported so far. Such supplements include gamma oryzanol (a plant sterol derived from rice bran oil), smilax, and yohimbine.

GINSENG SUPPLEMENTS Many people, including athletes, take ginseng supplements to boost their energy level. But studies carried out in 1996 and 1997 involving groups of people of average fitness showed no improvement in their metabolism or exercise performance while they were taking ginseng. The studies were conducted over periods of two to three months, however, so it is not known whether any benefits of ginseng might arise from long-term use.

FAT BURNERS IN THE MUSCLE CELLS

Some food supplements supposedly speed the rate at which fat passes into mitochondria, tiny powerhouses that are found in all cells, to be burned as energy. But this has not been proven scientifically. Mitochondria break down fatty acids and other food molecules to release energy. They are most numerous in the muscle cells that are highly active. The inner membranes of the mitochondria are folded to form shelves (cristae), and the spaces between the cristae contain the enzymes needed to break down fatty acids.

ENERGY CONVERSION
Muscle cells employed in aerobic activities contain thousands of mitochondria. Mitochondria use oxygen to convert fat into muscle energy.

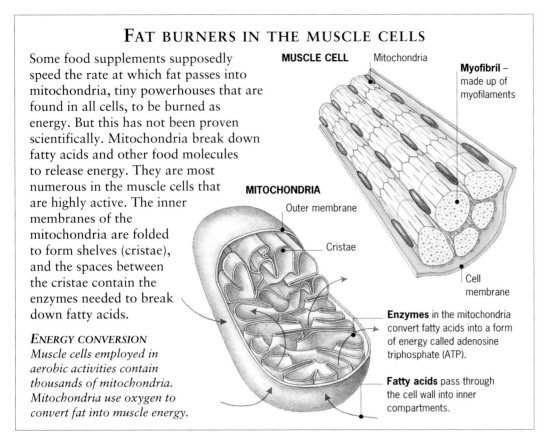

MUSCLE CELL — Mitochondria

Myofibril – made up of myofilaments

MITOCHONDRIA

Outer membrane

Cristae

Cell membrane

Enzymes in the mitochondria convert fatty acids into a form of energy called adenosine triphosphate (ATP).

Fatty acids pass through the cell wall into inner compartments.

Steroid abuse
In 1968 the International Olympic Committee banned the use of such performance-enhancing drugs as anabolic steroids by Olympic athletes and introduced drug testing. It is now known that many athletes under extreme pressure to succeed have used performance-enhancing drugs, despite their links to more than 70 health-damaging side effects. Anabolic steroids may still be used by some athletes during training, but the Olympic Committee now claims they can detect illegal drug use as far back as eight weeks.

VITAMINS AND MINERALS

Many exercisers believe that training can be improved by consuming vitamins in larger amounts than available in a normal diet. Vitamins and minerals do have an important role in the efficient functioning of the body, but taking large doses usually does not improve performance and can be harmful (see box, right).

There are a few exceptions. Some athletes are advised to take iron to keep their energy levels at their peak. (Always check with your doctor before taking an iron supplement.) Iron is an important constituent of the blood pigment in muscles and is a participant in energy-producing reactions of the body. Older persons and those who have disorders that prevent them from absorbing sufficient nutrients from food may also benefit from nutritional supplements.

FAT-MOBILIZING SUPPLEMENTS

Substances sold as "fat mobilizers" are said to break up fat and aid in its removal from the body, but at present no scientific evidence can back this claim. The only proven way to mobilize fat is to combine aerobic exercise with a low-fat diet. One substance sold as a fat-mobilizing agent is carnitine, which is needed for transporting fats into the mitochondria—microscopic structures that act as the powerhouse of each body cell (see box, above). The theory that carnitine can push more fats to be used as fuel is not supported. Inositol is another supposed fat mobilizer. But its value as a supplement is doubtful because it can be made in the body and is not a proven fat mobilizer. The same is true of lecithin, which emulsifies fats and aids digestion but does not promote fat loss.

VITAMIN LOADING AND MEGADOSES

When vitamins are taken in very large amounts, known as megadoses, they no longer function as vitamins but as drugs with medicinal actions. Evidence for the therapeutic effects of megadosing is still highly controversial.

The vitamins that have the most toxic effects when taken in excess are the fat-soluble ones—A, D, and to a lesser extent, E and K—which are easily stored in the body and can build up to harmful levels. The water-soluble vitamins, including the B complex and C, are thought to be less harmful because any excess is excreted by the body. However, it is believed that some B vitamins can lead to nerve disorders when taken in excess, and too much vitamin C can cause diarrhea and possibly kidney stones in susceptible people.

TONING UP YOUR SKIN

Although a daily regimen of cleansing and moisturizing goes a long way toward establishing a healthy complexion, the condition of your skin also reflects your lifestyle and diet.

The skin, the largest organ of the body, is the first line of defense in protecting the internal organs and muscles from damage and disease. It also regulates your body's temperature, increasing sweating if you get too hot and erecting the hair follicles (causing goose pimples) if you become cold. All people, regardless of age or sex, should look after their skin. The first step is to feed the skin from the inside with a healthy, balanced diet that is rich in vitamins and minerals. A routine of cleansing, exfoliating, toning, and moisturizing is also important, not just for women but for men as well. In addition, certain lifestyle factors, such as smoking and prolonged exposure to the sun, should be avoided in order to minimize damage to the skin.

THE STRUCTURE OF SKIN

The skin is made up of two main layers, the epidermis and the dermis, but it also has an underlying layer of subcutaneous tissue that is mostly adipose (fat) tissue.

The epidermis is the skin's protective layer. It contains rapidly dividing basal cells made up of a hard substance called keratin. New cells travel to the surface of the epidermis and die, forming a tough outer coating. As these cells wear away, they are replaced by new ones. Some cells produce the pigment melanin, which determines skin color; the more of these cells that are present, the darker the natural color of the skin.

The dermis is made up of connective tissue, including collagen and elastin, which together with subcutaneous fat are responsible for the skin's shape and elasticity. This layer houses hair follicles, sweat glands, and sebaceous glands, which produce the oily substance sebum. The dermis also houses the skin's sensory nerve endings, as well as blood and lymph vessels, which bring it nutrients and remove wastes.

SKIN TYPES

Sebum is the skin's natural lubricant; it keeps your hair and skin moisturized. If not enough is produced, the skin becomes very dry, while overproduction leads to oily skin.

HOW BLEMISHES DEVELOP

Each hair follicle contains a sebaceous gland that produces sebum, your body's own moisturizer, which keeps hair and skin supple. If excess sebum is produced, it can clog the opening to the hair follicle and trap bacteria inside. This causes the hair to die and a pimple to form. You can keep your pores clear with regular cleansing.

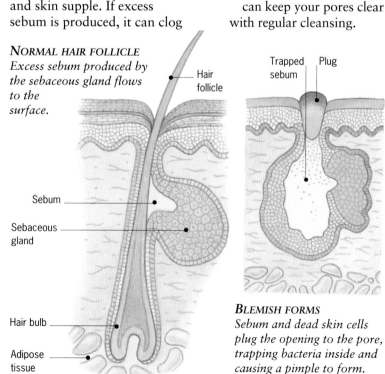

NORMAL HAIR FOLLICLE
Excess sebum produced by the sebaceous gland flows to the surface.

Hair follicle

Sebum

Sebaceous gland

Hair bulb

Adipose tissue

Trapped sebum   Plug

BLEMISH FORMS
Sebum and dead skin cells plug the opening to the pore, trapping bacteria inside and causing a pimple to form.

Knowing your skin type will help you to give it the proper care and avoid skin irritations and premature aging.

Dry skin: A fine, papery, or chalky texture is characteristic of dry skin; it also chaps easily and feels tight after washing. Regular moisturizing is important because the sebaceous glands do not produce enough oil to lubricate it well. Sebum declines with age, so it is even more important to moisturize this type of skin in later life.

Oily skin: Usually shiny and slightly greasy, oily skin often belongs to people with a sallow complexion and open pores. Because of an overproduction of sebum, the pores become clogged, causing pimples and blackheads. Regular cleansing is important to keep the pores clear. Teenagers often have oily skin due to an excess production of sex hormones. Most people develop fewer blemishes as they age because the level of sebum produced declines. For people who have oily skin throughout their lives there is some good news; oily skin stays free of wrinkles longer than any other type.

Combination skin: People with combination skin have both dry and oily patches. The oily patches tend to be in the T-shaped area of the forehead, nose, and chin, while the cheeks are dry. People with oily skin often develop combination skin as they age. Light moisturizing and the use of toning agents on oily areas will keep the skin clear.

Normal skin: Soft, with a supple texture and no dry or oily patches, normal skin is usually clear of blemishes, but it tends to become dry with age and is more likely to wrinkle. Light moisturizing after washing is all that is needed for normal skin until the dryness becomes more marked with passing time; then more intense moisturizing will be necessary.

EATING FOR HEALTHY SKIN

A varied diet that includes ample amounts of fruits, vegetables, seeds, and grains will be reflected in the glowing condition of your skin. But the first step toward a healthy complexion is to drink lots of liquid, at least eight glasses of water, juice, and other non-alcoholic and noncaffeinated beverages each day, to restore the body's fluid levels and flush toxins out of the system. Skin also needs a number of vitamins and minerals to keep it clear and smooth. The most important are the

DID YOU KNOW?
A 1963 study by American dermatologist Albert Kligman linked sun exposure to skin cancer and premature wrinkles. It was not until the early 1980s, two decades later, however, that ratings for the sun protection factor (SPF) were introduced for tanning products and cosmetics.

antioxidant vitamins, A, C, and E, and the mineral selenium. Antioxidants combat harmful free radicals, which are unstable molecules produced as a part of normal bodily processes and by pollution, sunlight, and cigarettes. They attack the cells, causing tissue damage and wrinkles. Antioxidants can be obtained from many plant sources, including fruits, particularly citrus fruits, berries, and melons, and brightly colored vegetables or leafy greens. They are also found in green tea.

SUMMER PUDDING

This recipe, packed with delicious fruits, is an excellent source of antioxidants, which feed your skin from the inside out.

15 medium-thick slices white bread, crusts removed
1½ lb mixed fruits, such as cherries, blackberries, raspberries, strawberries, and blueberries
1 tbsp sugar
mint sprigs for garnish
low-fat crème fraîche or sour cream for topping

■ Line six (6 oz) custard cups with 9 of the bread slices, cutting them to fit where necessary; do not overlap. (Reserve 6 bread slices to make the pudding lids.)
■ Wash the fruits. Hull and halve the strawberries. Remove stems and pits from the cherries.

■ Heat blueberries and cherries (if using) in a saucepan with the sugar and 5 tbsp of water over low heat. Cook, stirring, until fruit is tender. Remove from heat and add the remaining fruit, stirring gently to mix.
■ Spoon the fruit and most of the juice equally into the bread-lined custard cups, reserving a little juice to use later. Cut a lid for each pudding from the reserved bread slices. Put a weighted saucer on top of each pudding to keep the lids in place. Refrigerate the filled bowls on a tray to catch any overflowing juices.
■ Remove the weighted saucers and invert the puddings onto six serving plates. Spoon the reserved juices over them, garnish with mint sprigs, and serve with a dollop of crème fraîche or sour cream.
Serves 6

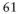

Skin Cleansers

Making your own skin cleansers from natural products not only saves you money but offers other benefits as well. For example, you will know that there are no additives to irritate sensitive skin and that the product hasn't been tested on animals.

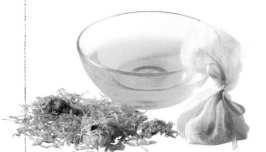

HERBAL INFUSION
If you prefer, use an herbal infusion instead of water for the cleanser below. Wrap 2 tablespoons of a dried herb, such as marigold, in muslin, pour boiling water over it, cover, and infuse for 10 minutes.

Each of the natural substances in these cleansers offers special properties that have particular benefits for the skin. For example, papaya contains a natural fruit acid, alpha hydroxy acid (AHA), that leaves the skin looking smoother and fresher, and papain, an enzyme that helps digest protein and remove dead skin cells. These properties give the complexion a healthy-looking glow and help dry out blemishes.

Homemade cleansers that do not include fresh ingredients will keep for about a month in an airtight container in the refrigerator.

BEESWAX AND ALMOND CLEANSING CREAM

This soft, fluffy cream is suitable for most skin types. Because wax is flammable, it should be heated slowly. The best way to do this is to use a hot-water bath, or *bain marie* (a bowl set over boiling water). This method heats the ingredients at the temperature of barely boiling water.

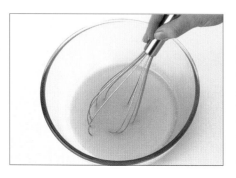

1 *Heat 25 g (1 oz) beeswax and ½ cup plus 2 tbsp almond oil in a water bath until the wax melts. In a small pan over low heat, bring ½ cup plus 2 tbsp water and ½ tsp borax to a simmer.*

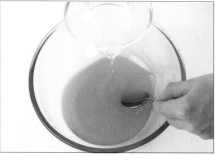

2 *Remove both containers from the heat. Stirring constantly, pour the water and borax mixture into the beeswax mixture. Continue to stir until the cream thickens and starts to cool.*

3 *Add about 10 drops of essential oil (see below for choices), beat the cream until cooled, and spoon into a dark-colored glass jar. Apply the cream with circular movements, using clean fingertips or a cotton pad. After about 30 seconds, remove with a tissue or dampened cotton pad or cotton ball. Essential oils, dry skin: jasmine, rose, lavender. Oily skin: geranium, bergamot, rosemary. Sensitive skin: chamomile.*

PAPAYA CLEANSER FOR PROBLEM SKIN

Cut a fully ripened papaya in half and remove the seeds. Scoop out the flesh and puree it in a blender or food processor until smooth. Apply the papaya to the face using gentle, circular movements. Leave for a few minutes and then wipe it off with a tissue and rinse with plenty of warm water.

GRAPEFRUIT CLEANSER FOR OILY SKIN

This cleanser is ideal if you enjoy grapefruit for breakfast. After eating your grapefruit, cut the empty shell into sections and rub the white fleshy sides in a circular motion all over your face. Leave the pulp for a few minutes, then rinse off with warm water and pat dry. Your skin will feel silky smooth.

Some foods should be avoided or consumed in moderation because they have a harmful effect on the skin. Excess amounts of saturated fat, for example, can cause an overproduction of free radicals in the body. They can also harm the lymph system, which has an important role to play in detoxifying the skin.

Tea, coffee, and alcohol, which increase fluid loss from the body through increased urination, cause dehydration. This reduces the skin's capacity to receive nutrients and remove toxins. Alcohol also depletes the body of B and C vitamins, thus promoting wrinkles and poor skin tone. Heavy alcohol consumption leads to facial flushing because alcohol dilates small blood vessels just below the surface of the skin; this condition can eventually become permanent.

Cigarettes and smoked, barbecued, or processed foods also increase levels of free radicals and reduce antioxidants in the body. Among other problems, this causes premature skin aging. Antioxidant supplements, especially vitamins C and E, can help to alleviate this but are no alternative to giving up smoking, moderating alcohol intake, and having a healthy and varied diet.

PREVENTING SKIN DAMAGE

Many of the threats to healthy skin come from the environment, both indoors and out. Exposure to excess sunlight, pollution, dry air, wind, rain, heat, cold, and cigarette smoke can all damage the skin.

Ultraviolet rays from the sun penetrate the dermis and break down collagen, even in winter, eventually causing sagging skin and wrinkles. Although a little exposure helps the body to produce vitamin D, sunlight that is strong enough to tan skin or cause peeling can age the skin prematurely. To keep a youthful complexion longer, it is advisable to protect your skin from bright sunlight year-round. Regularly apply a sunscreen with a sunburn prevention factor (SPF) of 15 or higher and wear a hat.

After sunlight, cigarette smoke has the most damaging effect on skin. Smokers have far more wrinkles than nonsmokers and often have a pale, gray, or sallow complexion. Their skin is also thicker and may have broken veins. Because smoking depletes vitamin C in the body, skin damage heals at a slower rate. Eating foods rich in vitamin C or taking a supplement can help offset the damage, but smoking's effect on the skin is yet another reason, along with increased well-being and a reduced risk of major diseases, for giving it up altogether.

Central heating and air conditioning produce an arid atmosphere that quickly dries the skin. You can counteract this by using a humidifier or placing a bowl of water by a radiator to add moisture to the air. Cold wind also dries the skin, so use moisturizer regularly to compensate. Sudden changes in temperature—going out into the cold from a warm room, for example—can cause delicate blood vessels in the skin to burst, resulting in thread (spider) veins on the cheeks and nose. To avoid this, lower the room temperature or move to a cooler room to give your body time to adjust before going outside.

THE AGING PROCESS

Skin has a built-in biological clock in its cells that determines how and when it will age. This natural, inevitable process varies for each of us, depending on our genetic inheritance. Look at your parents to see how their skin has aged, and you will get a good idea of what will happen to you.

Starting at about age 30, the plump, unwrinkled skin of youth begins to change. The cells no longer renew themselves as readily, and other functions of the skin, such as oil production, begin to slow down. At the same time the skin loses its flexibility as a result of reduced collagen production. With advancing age, the skin's outer layer becomes thinner, making it less resistant to damage. It also loses some of its elasticity, and wrinkles begin to appear.

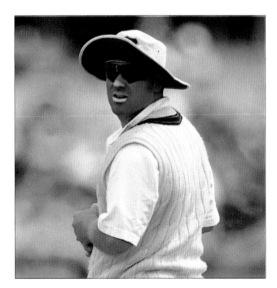

SKIN CARE FOR SPORTS Sensible sun precautions, shown here on Australian cricketer Shane Warne, include a hat to keep the sun off the face and the back of the neck, sunglasses to protect the eyes, and total sunblock on sensitive areas such as the nose and lips. If possible, use waterproof sun products because sweat from exertion can quickly wash other types away. Reapply a cream regularly.

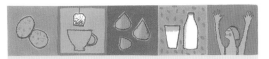

SUPER SHAPER

Cleopatra knew a good beauty product —milk—when she bathed in it. Milk protein has the same effect when applied to skin as when it is drunk; it builds, repairs, and reconditions. The lactic acid base can actually reinforce the skin's natural acid mantle, which protects against the harmful effects of bacteria, alcohol, smoke, sun, and wind, and helps to maintain the skin's pH balance. Milk is an increasingly popular ingredient in beauty products, which include milk baths, milk soap bars, and milk shampoos. In fact, milk can be used directly from the bottle to effectively cleanse and nourish the skin.

In addition to genetic factors and natural aging, your skin is subjected to a number of damaging forces, including sunlight, wind, and excessive heat and cold. Environmental pollution, such as car exhaust fumes, background radiation, and other toxic emissions, can also take their toll. Sometimes the skin has an allergic reaction to such substances as medications and cosmetics. Skin also reacts adversely to emotional stress, lack of exercise, sleep deprivation, and sometimes to fluctuating hormone levels.

Exercise and skin problems

Although exercise is excellent for the skin, it can foster some problems. Sweat, if left on the skin, can promote the breeding of bacteria that cause body odor. These bacteria live on the skin's surface, and when sweat comes into contact with them, an unpleasant odor occurs. This odor takes a few hours to develop, however, so if you wash regularly and use an antiperspirant, it should not be a problem. If you suffer from excessive sweating, you may need to see your doctor for a stronger prescription antiperspirant.

There are other skin problems caused indirectly by exercise, the most common being the fungal infection athlete's foot. It breeds freely in warm, damp conditions such as shower rooms and produces an itchy, red rash and flaking skin between the toes and on the soles of the feet. The skin may crack, leading to painful open sores. People with sweaty feet are more prone to athlete's foot. Topical antifungal creams and powders are available to kill fungi and prevent them from growing. For persistent cases a doctor may prescribe antifungal tablets to be taken for about three months.

Chlorine in swimming pools can also irritate sensitive skin. There is a trend toward lowering the amount of chlorine in pool water, which may help reduce the discomfort, and you can look for a facility that advertises this approach. Always shower thoroughly after swimming and soothe skin with chamomile cream.

Blisters can develop from ill-fitting sports shoes; they are very painful but usually clear up once the shoes are replaced and the blisters have burst naturally. (You should never open a blister yourself.)

SKIN CLEANSERS

The skin is covered with cavities in which dirt, grime, oil, and dead skin cells accumulate, leading to blemishes and blackheads. Cleansing the skin first thing in the morning and last thing at night removes impurities and allows the skin to breathe. There are several types of cleanser to choose from.

Soap: Because soap is usually alkaline, it can irritate the skin, which has a slightly acidic composition. Some soaps include moisturizers and are not as alkaline; these are generally kinder to the skin.

Cream cleansers: Usually intended for use on the face, cream cleansers contain emulsifiers to dissolve dirt particles and makeup. Rich, creamy types should be lightly massaged over the skin, while thinner ones should be applied and then removed with a tissue.

Liquid cleansers: Whether a liquid cleanser is milky or creamy, apply it lightly to the face, then remove it with tissue or a cotton pad.

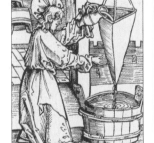

AN ANCIENT ART
This woodcut showing the making of lye, a liquid solution of potash essential for soap making, dates from 1514. It is not known exactly when soap was first made, but it may have been as far back as prehistoric times. The earliest record we have for soap making is from the Babylonians around 2800 B.C.

DID YOU KNOW?

According to ancient Roman legend, the word *soap* was derived from Mount Sapo, a place where animals were sacrificed. Rain washed a mixture of animal fat, or tallow, and wood ashes down into the clay soil along the River Tiber. Women who washed their clothes in the river found that using this clay mixture made their wash cleaner.

Moisturizers

Moisturizers help skin to recover from day-to-day damage. If you use fresh natural ingredients to make your own, any active constituents, such as vitamins, minerals, and essential fatty acids, will be more effective.

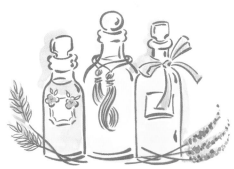

Homemade moisturizers can often be more effective than store-bought products. Most will last about a month, but this time may be reduced to just a few days if fresh ingredients are used. You should avoid the eyelids when applying moisturizer and always test a small amount of a new product on your inner elbow or wrist before applying it elsewhere, particularly if you have sensitive or allergy-prone skin.

PRESENTING HOMEMADE PRODUCTS
Select attractive, airtight glass jars or ceramic pots for your products. With simple decoration, they can be presented as a special gift with a personal touch.

AVOCADO AND HONEY CREAM FOR DRY OR OLDER SKINS

Skin that lacks moisture needs a good skin lubricant, like avocado. This fruit contains plant oils that are rich in essential fatty acids—particularly linoleic acid. These not only serve as natural moisturizers but also strengthen the membranes that surround skin cells. You should store this cream in the refrigerator and use it within three days.

• Using a food processor, blender, wire masher, or mortar and pestle, mash half a ripe avocado until smooth and lump free. You may need to push it through a sieve to make it smooth.
• Add 1 tbsp honey or olive oil and a drop of calendula essential oil; stir the ingredients until completely combined. If you have spider veins or sensitive, mature, or wrinkled skin, you can substitute neroli essential oil for the calendula.

PEPPERMINT AND TEA TREE CREAM FOR OILY SKIN

Oily skin does need moisturizing, but products with a high oil content should be avoided. This cream includes jojoba oil, which closely matches the skin's own oil, or sebum, making it ideal for oily skin. It also includes tea tree oil, which has an antiseptic quality and is an effective treatment for acne-prone skin.

• In a bowl set in a hot-water bath (see page 62), melt 11 g (⅓ oz) grated beeswax with 4 tsp jojoba oil. Meanwhile, prepare 3 fl oz (⅓ cup) of peppermint tea. Add ½ tsp borax to the hot tea.
• Remove the wax from the heat and slowly trickle in the tea, whisking constantly with a wire whisk or electric mixer until an emulsion has formed.
• Cool slightly, then blend 8 drops peppermint and 4 drops tea tree oil into the mixture, stirring to combine.

RICH CITRUS NIGHT CREAM FOR ALL SKIN TYPES

This cream can be made easily from ingredients that are readily available. Because the ingredients are fresh, it will last about a week. Apply the cream with clean fingers and wipe off any excess with tissue or a cotton pad after about 20 minutes.

• Mix ½ tsp freshly squeezed lemon juice and 1 tsp freshly squeezed orange juice in a medium-size bowl.
• Add 3 egg yolks and 1 tsp glycerin to the juice and beat with a whisk until well combined.
• Drizzle 2 to 3 tsp olive oil very slowly into the mixture, beating all the time, until the mixture is thick.
• Beat in 1 to 2 tbsp plain yogurt to thin the mixture to the desired consistency.

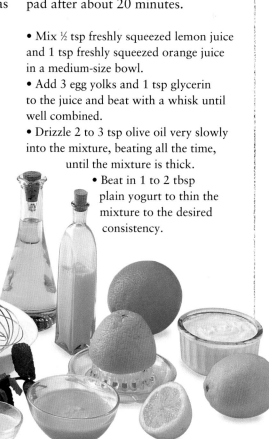

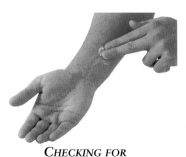

CHECKING FOR SENSITIVITY
Even if you do not think you have sensitive skin, it is always best to test a new product, whether homemade or store-bought. Place a small amount on an area of sensitive skin, such as the inside of the wrist or elbow, and leave it for 5 minutes. If there is no reaction, you can safely apply it more freely.

Water-soluble cleansers: Usually applied to damp skin and massaged in, water-soluble cleansers wash off with warm water.

Gel or oil cleansers: A gel or oil cleanser is massaged onto slightly damp skin and rinsed off with warm water. Some have antiseptic properties to help combat blemishes.

Body washes and shower gels: Used as a substitute for soap, mainly in the shower, body washes and gels are massaged over the skin and then rinsed off under the shower.

CLEANSERS FOR DIFFERENT SKIN TYPES

Each type of cleanser suits different kinds of skin. A creamy cleanser is most appropriate for removing makeup and daily grime from dry and older skin—soap is too astringent. A toner lotion should then be used to remove any traces of the cleanser. Rinse your face in water afterward only if you have soft water. Hard water contains mineral deposits that can accumulate on skin.

You can use a mild soap if you have oily or combination skin, but it is best to use a cleansing lotion first to remove makeup. Medicated soaps are suitable for patches that are prone to blemishes but should not be used on any dry areas because they can cause scaling. Mild soaps or cleansing lotions are fine if you have normal skin. However, you may need to try different products to find one that works well for your particular complexion. Whatever agent you use, your night cleansing routine should be more rigorous in order to remove the daily accumulation of dirt and makeup.

MOISTURIZERS

Because environmental conditions, cleansing, and advancing age can deplete your skin of water, a moisturizer should be applied regularly to replenish the loss. Many daytime moisturizers now include sun protection and soothing herbal extracts that help to combat skin irritations as well. The best time to apply a moisturizer is right after washing or showering, when the skin is already hydrated.

Moisturizers are available in a variety of formulations for various types of skin and different parts of the body. A lighter moisturizer suits normal, combination, and oily skins. A richer one is better for dry skin. Night moisturizing creams tend to be richer and are designed to work throughout the

---

ALOE VERA AND COCONUT SHAVING CREAM

This shaving cream is ideal for a man's beard or for women to use on legs and underarms. The emollient properties of coconut soothe the skin, while the healing aloe vera gel deals with any razor nicks. Natural plant oils leave the skin silky smooth, and there is no need to use an additional moisturizer after shaving. Store in an airtight tub and use within one month. After shaving, remove excess cream with a warm damp cloth and pat the skin dry.

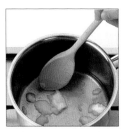

1 *Melt 175 g (6 oz) coconut oil over low heat. When liquid, remove from the heat and whisk in 2 tsp witch hazel and 50 ml (2 tbsp) almond oil.*

3 *To shave, rub a clump of cream in the hands until liquid. Apply an even layer to the skin, adding more as necessary.*

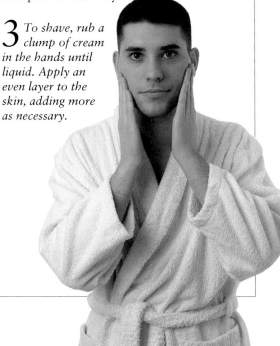

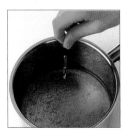

2 *Whisk in 1 tbsp aloe vera gel until combined. Leave to cool slightly, then add 8 drops lavender essential oil. Leave in the refrigerator until set.*

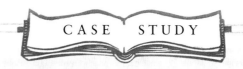
A Middle-aged Acne Sufferer

A good diet and regular exercise go hand in hand to create a healthy body and mind. However, too much exercise can suppress the immune system, and when the diet is wrong too, this combination can lead to skin problems. Emotional factors affect the physical body as well. If both body and mind are under stress, other physical problems may develop.

Gwen is a 44-year-old part-time dental nurse. After her divorce three years ago, she joined a health club, working out regularly on the gym machines, taking step-aerobics classes, and playing tennis.

Although her complexion has always been fairly clear, Gwen has had occasional blemishes on her face, back, and chest. Recently they have become worse, and she has also developed a skin infection between her thighs and under her breasts.

Gwen went to see a dermatologist, who identified her infection as a fungal disease and recommended an antifungal cream. He also prescribed a retinol-based cream for her blemishes and advised her to see a dietitian, who will analyze her diet to see if it is adequate.

WHAT SHOULD GWEN DO?

Gwen should use the acne and anti-fungal creams as prescribed, and her skin will gradually improve. She should also follow through on the advice to see a dietitian; since the divorce, she has not been eating as regularly and she often does not prepare herself an evening meal.

Because Gwen was devastated by her divorce and has found being alone hard to deal with, she should investigate whether her skin problems could be linked to emotional difficulties. Suppressed emotions and the stress of dramatic lifestyle changes can affect the immune system, leaving the body more prone to infections. Too much intense exercise can also have a detrimental effect on immune function.

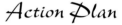

Action Plan

DIET
Establish a regular eating pattern, reduce saturated fat and sugar, and eat more fruits and vegetables to purify the skin and boost the immune system.

EXERCISE
Temporarily reduce exercise levels to allow the body to direct its energy toward strengthening the immune system.

EMOTIONAL HEALTH
Seek help from a counselor to solve deep-rooted emotional conflicts that may be the cause of the skin problems.

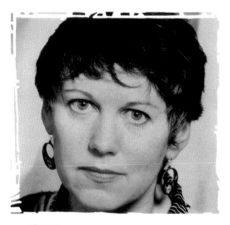

EMOTIONAL HEALTH
Excessive activity can often be a way of avoiding emotional conflicts that need to be tackled.

DIET
A diet low in fruits and vegetables but high in fats and sugar suppresses the immune system and creates an environment in which infection can thrive.

EXERCISE
Moderate exercise can aid the immune system, but when taken to excess, it can reduce the body's ability to fight off infection.

HOW THINGS TURNED OUT FOR GWEN

Gwen used the prescribed creams religiously and reduced her activities to sessions of tennis and aerobics. She consulted a dietitian, who helped her devise a healthful diet plan, and she has stuck with it. She also saw a counselor, who helped her to deal with her suppressed emotions.

Gwen is feeling healthier and much more optimistic now that she is dealing positively with both her physical and her emotional problems.

night. They are most suitable for dry and older skins; people with oily, combination, or normal skins may find a daytime moisturizer just as effective for night use. Nighttime moisturizers are said to contain ingredients that feed the skin as you sleep, but many of the claims are largely unproven.

Some creams are too heavy for the delicate skin around the eyes and may cause irritation, so special creams have been devised for this area. Many eye creams also help reduce puffiness, minimize shadows, and reduce fine lines.

Hands need regular applications of moisturizer because they are constantly exposed to air, frequent washing, and contact with household chemicals. A layer of hand cream restores moisture and soothes the skin.

The skin on your body also needs moisturizing because bathing and showering remove oils. People who exercise tend to take more showers and so need extra skin care. Body lotions are lighter and more readily absorbed than face creams, both for convenience and because the body skin is less exposed than the face and thus does not require rich preparations.

Antiaging creams

Antiaging creams and lotions tighten the skin, minimizing the appearance of fine lines, and rehydrate the top layer of cells, making the skin look smoother and more pliant. Creams containing retinoic acid (a form of vitamin A) gradually remove layers of skin to reduce lines. Retinoic acid was used only to treat acne for a number of years, but scientific trials showed that it can help reverse photoaging—the premature aging of the skin caused by the sun. Retinoic acid can cause side effects, such as flaking, dryness, and reddening, and must be prescribed by a doctor.

Alpha hydroxy acids (AHAs), which occur naturally in many fruits, vegetables, and milk, are added to some moisturizers. They work by loosening the protein that glues the surface cells together, thus removing the outer layers of skin, accelerating cell renewal, and unblocking clogged pores. These actions make the skin appear smoother and less lined. A high AHA level can cause reddening and flaking. If you have sensitive skin, choose a lower one; most products range from 1 to 10 percent AHA. Stronger concentrations are available by prescription to treat acne.

SKIN TREATMENTS

The skin is constantly under assault from makeup, pollution, central heating, air conditioning, and hormonal changes. This assault can leave it looking tired, drawn, sallow, and in need of a pick-me-up. There is a range of beauty treatments that aim to cleanse, moisturize, and revitalize the skin. Although the health claims made for some treatments are unproven, there is evidence that regular beauty care with such products keeps the skin clear, hydrated, and blemish-free and helps reduce fine lines.

Masks (face packs): Applied to cleansed, moist skin, masks remove dead skin cells and impurities, open the pores, and stimulate circulation, making the skin smoother. The mask is left on for 10 to 15 minutes and then removed. There are two types of mask: mud packs, which are washed off, and gel-like products, which harden and must be peeled off. After removal of a mask, the skin should be rinsed with toner, and with the exception of very oily skin, a moisturizer should be applied.

Exfoliants (scrubs): Containing gritty materials, exfoliants are massaged over the face to remove outer layers of epidermal cells and stimulate cell renewal to make the skin look

---

NATURAL FACE SCRUB

This face scrub of natural products removes dead skin cells, encourages the growth of new cells, feeds the skin, and improves blood circulation and lymphatic drainage. The recipe makes enough for two applications.

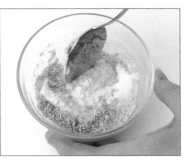

1 *In a small bowl, mix 1 tbsp grapefruit juice, 2 tbsp ground oatmeal, and ½ tbsp plain yogurt until well combined into a paste.*

2 *Smooth the mixture over the face, working it well into the skin. Leave for 10 minutes and then rinse off with warm water.*

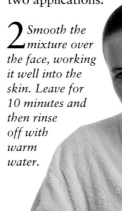

THERAPEUTIC MUD BATHS

Mud baths work on the same principle as face packs but are applied to the whole body. Special types of mud rich in vitamins, minerals, and other elements are said to have therapeutic properties, as well as the ability to remove impurities from the skin. Therapeutic mud baths are popular in continental Europe, but there are mud spas throughout the world. Depending on where the mud comes from, its active constituents vary. Therapeutic mud is used to treat such conditions as arthritis and rheumatism, skin disorders, reproductive disorders, and digestive problems, including stomach ulcers. One famous therapeutic mud is found in Neydharting, Australia, and is exported worldwide for beauty treatments.

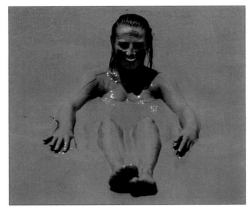

VOLCANIC SUPERMUD
Natural mud baths are found in countries with thermal or volcanic activity (often the same country has both). The volcanic mud naturally occurring in Arborettes, Colombia (above), is believed to have healing powers.

and feel fresher and smoother. Some exfoliants work by loosening surface cells with chemicals rather than abrasive substances.

Steaming: A deep-cleansing treatment, steaming helps soften the skin, reduce oiliness, unblock pores, and loosen blackheads. It is unsuitable for anyone who is prone to spider veins on the face because the heat dilates blood vessels in the skin.

To give yourself a steam treatment, pour boiling water into a bowl and add a few drops of essential oil suitable to your skin type (see page 62), stirring well. Lean over the bowl with a towel draped over your head and around the bowl to keep the steam enclosed. Remain in this position for 5 to 10 minutes to allow the warm vapors to loosen dirt and cleanse the pores.

A full facial: Available at beauty salons and spas, a facial combines various face treatments tailored to your skin type. First, makeup is removed, the skin is thoroughly cleansed, and the cleanser is removed with toner. The face may then be steamed, with the eyes protected with pads steeped in a lotion to reduce puffiness. The next stage may be a moisturizing mask or exfoliation, depending on skin type. Moisturizing cream is then massaged into the face and neck, using sweeping upward movements.

A face massage: A face massage can help to reduce fine lines on the face and relax tensed facial muscles, especially when it is done with lubricating oils or moisturizers. For a home massage, rub a little massage oil on your fingertips and, starting on the inner eyebrows, make gentle, circular movements. Work your way up to the forehead, across the temples, down the cheekbones, across the nose, and down to the chin. Repeat, reversing the sequence.

Body massage: Massage is beneficial for the whole body, especially when combined with aromatherapy—the application of massage oil that contains essential oils, which are absorbed through the pores. Aromatherapy massage can relieve stress, migraines, tension headaches, muscle strains, and menstrual and circulatory problems. Relaxing oils are frankincense, ylang ylang, neroli, and myrrh. Stimulating oils include all of the citrus family, plus peppermint, pine, and basil. For muscle strains, cypress, hyssop, marjoram, and black pepper are recommended. Oils to relieve menstrual problems include geranium, chamomile, and jasmine. Circulatory problems can be eased with juniper, clary sage, and ginger.

Body wrap: The body may be covered with such substances as seaweed, herbs, or algae and then wrapped in warm towels to encourage the active constituents to be absorbed into the skin. It is claimed that some components of the plant material break down fat and water deposits, helping to detoxify the body and improve skin tone.

Turkish baths
Originating in the Middle East, Turkish baths have been established in America since the 19th century. The main feature of a Turkish bath is a room filled with hot moist air, where clients may relax or have a massage. To prepare the body for massage, customers sit in a sauna, then plunge into a cold-water pool, alternating between the two extremes a few times.

The heat of the sauna and steam room opens the pores to aid removal of toxins and excess fluid from body tissues. A Turkish bath may help relieve conditions like fluid retention, joint and muscle pain, and stress. People with circulatory or heart disorders should check with a doctor before having a Turkish bath.

FRUIT AND VEGETABLE SKIN BOOSTERS

Eating at least five servings of fruits and vegetables every day will not only keep your skin in better condition but can also help it to fight problems like dryness and acne. Many fruits and vegetables are particularly good sources of the antioxidant vitamins A and C, bioflavonoids, and the mineral potassium. The antioxidants neutralize harmful free radicals created by pollution and the body's metabolic processes. Vitamin C is used by the skin also to make collagen, a protein that maintains its flexibility and strength. Bioflavonoids help to stabilize collagen and maintain a barrier against harmful bacteria and skin inflammation. Potassium is vital for controlling water balance in the body's tissues and cells.

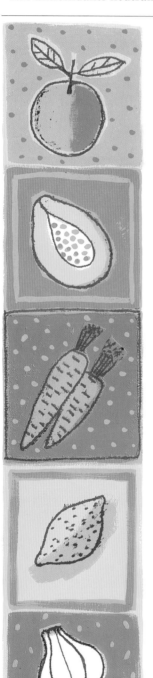

APPLES

Apples contain good amounts of both soluble and insoluble dietary fiber, which speeds the body's elimination of waste products and thus helps to keep the skin clear.

AVOCADOS

Rich in the antioxidant vitamins, A, C, and E, and in vitamins B_6, folic acid, niacin, magnesium, and potassium, avocados are also widely used in commercial skin preparations.

BEETS

Beets are high in folic acid, iron, and potassium and contain a fair amount of calcium. Their green tops are especially rich in the antioxidant vitamins A and C.

CARROTS

Carrots are a very rich source of beta carotene, the precursor to vitamin A; one carrot can provide as much as two to three times the recommended daily allowance of this antioxidant.

GARLIC

Garlic has antiseptic, antibacterial, antiviral, and antifungal properties. It is a natural detoxifier and antioxidant that strengthens the immune system.

SEAWEED

Seaweed is a good source of calcium, potassium, iron, magnesium, iodine, and zinc, which can help keep the complexion clear. However, you must eat a large serving to reap the benefits.

MELONS

All melons are low in calories and high in water content, which helps keep the skin hydrated. Most are good sources of vitamin C and potassium, and the orange varieties contain vitamin A.

PARSLEY

Parsley is rich in vitamin C and iron, also contains calcium, magnesium, phosphorus, potassium, and chlorophyll, and has traces of zinc and manganese.

PEPPERS

Peppers, both sweet and hot, have very high levels of vitamin C. They are also rich in beta carotene, iron, and potassium, all of which are good skin protectors.

WATERCRESS

Watercress, like other dark leafy greens, is a good source of vitamins A and C. It also contains bioflavonoids, which work alongside antioxidants in preventing cell damage.

PINEAPPLE

The inside of a pineapple makes an ideal exfoliant when rubbed over the skin. Pineapple is also good in facial treatments for problem skin. When eaten, it is a good source of vitamin C.

PAPAYAS

An excellent source of vitamins A, C, and folic acid, papayas are also a good skin-care product because they contain the fruit enzyme papain, which can be used to exfoliate and heal skin.

BANANAS

Bananas contain good levels of a wide range of vitamins and minerals, including potassium and vitamin C; they are used in many natural skin-care products as well.

LEMONS

Along with other citrus fruits, lemons are good sources of vitamin C. When applied to skin, lemon juice softens it and aids in removing the residues of soap and hard water.

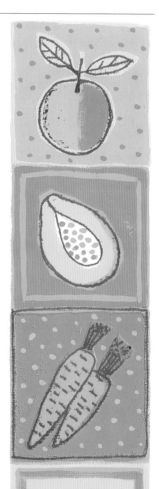
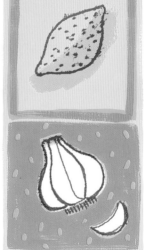

MATCHING YOUR STYLE TO YOUR SHAPE

Your personal style, reflected in your choice of clothes and hairstyle, can play an important role in enhancing your shape and accentuating your best features.

Although diet and exercise can alter overall appearance, your essential shape—the structure of your bones and muscles and distribution of your body fat—will be largely unchanged throughout your life. The way you dress can help you make the most of your natural assets and draw attention away from problem areas. Other factors, however, such as wearing high heels or carrying bags incorrectly, can cause bad posture and misalignment in the body.

THE IMPORTANCE OF UNDERWEAR

What you wear underneath your clothes can make a difference in your shape and overall appearance. Many large department stores offer a free fitting service with staff trained to give advice and assistance on choosing the right undergarments.

A properly fitted bra is an important influence on a woman's posture and appearance. The suspensory ligaments that support the breasts stretch naturally with time, allowing the breasts to sag. A bra lends support to these ligaments and helps keep the breasts firm and well shaped. Wearing a bra is especially important during exercise, when strenuous movement puts the suspensory ligaments under extra strain, creating a greater risk of stretching. A strong, well-fitting sports bra prevents this problem by holding the breasts securely in place.

Ill-fitting bras can throw the body out of balance, causing bad posture. If the straps of the bra are too tight, for example, they can put pressure on the shoulder blades and the base of the neck—a problem most often found in large-breasted women. The shoulders may also push back to compensate for a lack of support or hunch over to hide the fact that a bra accentuates a large bust.

Figure-shaping undergarments

Support garments can improve shape by pulling in the waist and flattening the stomach, but most have drawbacks. They can restrict the body's natural functions, such as breathing and digestion. If the back muscles come to rely too much on the support provided by a corset, the spine can become seriously weakened as well. Also, the abdominal muscles can lose tone through habitual wearing of a girdle, which in turn can lead

THE ROLE OF THE SUSPENSORY LIGAMENTS

A woman's breasts are supported by strips of connective tissue called suspensory ligaments. These ligaments are connected to the muscles of the underarm, shoulders, and chest, all of which are a vital part of the breast support structure. Exercises that tone and strengthen the muscles will help to maintain firm breasts.

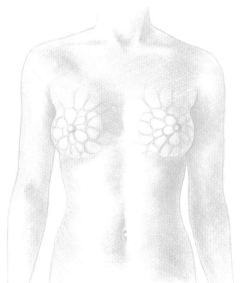

BREAST SLING
The breast ligaments form a slinglike arrangement that gives them support. However, this sling is inelastic; once it becomes stretched and the breasts drop, they cannot return to their former position. A bra provides vital support and should be worn throughout life, starting with the onset of puberty, when the breasts start to gain in size and weight. An extra-supportive bra is needed when ligaments are under increased strain, such as when playing a sport or breast-feeding.

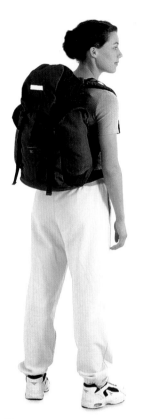

*DISTRIBUTING WEIGHT
EVENLY
Carrying a heavy bag on
one shoulder can throw
your back out of align-
ment, leading to back,
shoulder, and neck
problems. The best way
to distribute any weight
you carry evenly is to use
a backpack, correctly
fitted with padded straps
over both shoulders.
If you do use a hand-
bag, choose one that has
a shoulder strap and
bring the strap across the
body from the opposite
shoulder and change
shoulders often.*

to sagging and a buildup of fat. In addition, support garments do not solve the problem of excess fat but simply relocate it, often producing bulges in other areas of the body. It is much better to challenge weight problems with exercise and dietary measures before resorting to figure-shaping undergarments, although, as with high heels, occasional wear does little harm.

SHOES

No part of your outfit will dictate the way you look and feel as much as your footwear. Good foot support is particularly important during exercise. A wide selection of exercise footwear is available, and it is advisable to seek advice in choosing the right shoe for the activity you will be doing. A shoe meant for tennis, for example, differs from one designed for aerobics. For day-to-day living, wear comfortable shoes that fit well but do not pinch. Women should avoid high heels on a regular basis and wear flat shoes or ones with a slightly raised heel; the latter allows ease of movement but offers a small lift to flatter your legs.

High heels and a woman's shape

In general, women like wearing high heels and men like to see women wearing them. This is because they make the legs appear longer and the feet smaller—both considered attractive characteristics. They also distort the posture, pushing the pelvis forward and forcing the lower back to arch and the buttocks and belly to stick out. The effect may be sexually enticing, but the distortion to the spine and posture can be damaging. When you wear high heels, your weight is balanced on the ball of the foot, which causes instability and weakening of the joints and muscles, especially in the ankle and lower back. Your toes are also squeezed against the front of the shoes, which can cause bunions and other malformations.

ACCESSORIES

Accessories, particularly belts, can enhance and flatter your shape. Women often use such items as scarves and shawls, jewelry, hats, handbags, gloves, and glasses to set off their outfits, but it is important that they not allow accessories to overwhelm their appearance. In general, small accessories are a better choice for petite women and larger accessories look better on large ladies.

Belts can be used to draw in the waist and emphasize the body's shape, but people who lack much waistline, having either a very rounded or a straight figure, should avoid drawing attention to the waist with a belt. Women with well-defined waistlines, especially those with larger hips and busts, benefit from wearing a narrow belt.

Shoulder pads in women's clothes and shoulder reinforcements in men's suits and jackets provide lift and can help balance the structure of a person's figure. They can also take the emphasis away from a thickening waistline or large stomach. Shoulder pads balance the shape of women who have a fuller figure or large bust, but they should be avoided by anyone with large or square shoulders; they will result in a top-heavy look. Women should avoid wearing both a dress and a jacket with shoulder pads because this will exaggerate the shoulders.

Women can also use scarves and shawls to accentuate the shoulders, drawing attention away from a large bust or stomach.

Bags, handbags, and backpacks

To avoid developing aches in the back and shoulders, consider the effect on your posture of different handbags and the way you carry them. A single bag unbalances the body by altering the center of gravity, pulling one side down and putting the shoulders out of alignment, whereas a backpack distributes the weight evenly on both shoulders (see far left column). No matter what kind of bag you use, limit the contents. According to experts, women carry far too much in their handbags—12 pounds is recommended as the maximum weight to carry on a regular basis.

Carrying shopping bags properly can also prevent strain and pain. You should change hands often; better yet, distribute the contents in two bags.

IMPROVING YOUR SHAPE WITH STYLE MANAGEMENT

Using clothing and style tricks to emphasize your best features and hide your worst can make a big difference in your appearance. Look at your body in a mirror and decide, as objectively as you can, which features you want to emphasize and which parts you would rather conceal.

You can then work on different combinations of clothes to find the balance that suits you. Different clothing styles complement certain shapes and work against others. Men who have a classic inverted triangle shape, for example, may appear top-heavy in a long jacket or a coat with padded shoulders. Wearing a softer look that avoids the emphasis on the shoulders can balance the shape better. They should avoid tight-fitting shirts that accentuate their muscular shoulders and chest. Wearing an open neckline will break a wide shoulder line, making it appear smaller, and tucking shirts in at the waist will help prevent a stocky appearance. Loose, pleated trousers will give the lower part of the body more bulk.

Playing down height

Tall people often feel that they stand out too much, and they may try to compensate by stooping, which is bad for the back. It is much better to balance your tall figure with well-chosen clothes. Wear jackets that cover your buttocks (shorter jackets exaggerate height) but avoid long coats. Using several different colors or patterns in your outfit will break up your silhouette and help reduce your apparent height. Tall women benefit from wearing loose-fitting pants and fuller dresses. Knee-length skirts reduce leg length, especially when worn with a long, loose-fitting blouse or tunic. Tall men look best in well-fitted trousers that are neither too tight nor too loose.

Disguising the stomach

A common dilemma is how to disguise a large stomach. Drawing attention to another part of the body is one of the best strategies. Men should choose longer jackets with padded shoulders; these help hide the abdomen and draw attention to the shoulders instead. Pants with pleats help to balance the abdomen and legs, evening out proportions. Loose-fitting shirts and tops tucked into the pants camouflage stomach size.

Plumper or well-rounded women should aim to extend their overall length by drawing attention to the legs, face, and neckline and away from the waist. V-necks, scarves,

DRESSING FOR YOUR AGE

How you dress has a significant effect on how you look, feel, and are perceived. Here are tips to avoid looking at odds with who you really are.

▶ *Older men and women should avoid mixing lots of bright colors.*

▶ *Unless they have the figure for it, women should avoid wearing very short or very tight dresses or skirts.*

▶ *Strappy or strapless dresses are meant for women with toned upper bodies, not flabby arms or loose skin.*

▶ *Don't get locked into a time zone that is long gone. Keep an eye on current fashions and update or get rid of items that are outdated. You can't go wrong building your wardrobe on classic styles that never go out of fashion.*

FLATTER YOUR BODY SHAPE

Although diet and exercise can help you to lose weight and tone your body, your basic shape will remain unchanged. This is where clothes can play a useful role in helping you to look in proportion. The right outfit will emphasize your best points, as well as draw attention away from problem areas.

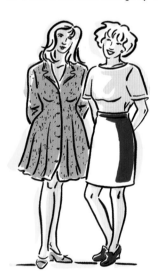 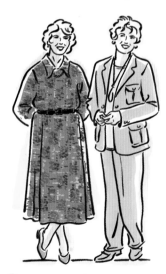 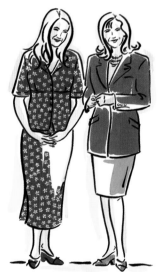

LARGE HIPS
Wear darker colors and plain colors or vertical stripes on your lower half. Pleats, bulky fabrics, and outfits with a nipped-in waist will make your hips look bigger.

ROUNDED SHAPE
Choose clothes that elongate your figure, such as tailored jackets with small shoulder pads. Avoid details like belts, pleats, or gathers that draw attention to the waist.

TALL WOMEN
To avoid looking taller than you are, avoid long skirts or dresses with small or fussy patterns. Opt for outfits in bold colors and wear more dramatic accessories.

Hair and your shape

Hairstyle is an integral part of your personal appearance. Follow these simple guidelines for a style that complements the shape of your face:

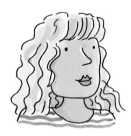

SQUARE FACE
Soften the lines of a square face by framing it with bangs and curls or long waves at the sides.

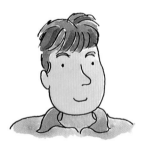

ROUND FACE
Choose a style that is shorter at the sides but full at the crown to give more length to the face.

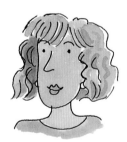

LONG FACE
A wavy style that is full at the sides but short at the crown helps to balance a long face.

soft collars, and necklaces draw attention to and complement the face and neckline. Long, loose-fitting jackets, blouses, and tunics, especially with padded shoulders, help even out proportions. Knee-length skirts will draw the eye to the legs, but shorts should be avoided. Both sexes with rounded figures should choose plain patterns and muted colors and avoid stripes and checks, which accentuate shape.

Increasing stature

Tall, thin men sometimes look shapeless and lacking in substance. Clothes that provide shape can help to offset this effect. It is important that garments not be baggy, however, as this tends to give the impression of your being too small for the clothes. Padded shoulders will fill out the upper half of the body and better define the shoulders. Well-fitted pants will also give the body a better definition. Baggy or pleated pants should be avoided. When choosing fabrics, it is best to avoid vertical stripes, which make the body appear taller and leaner; horizontal stripes have the opposite effect. V-necklines and open shirt collars tend to elongate the face, making it look thinner; round-necked tops are a better choice.

The most important rule for petite women is to wear well-fitted clothes that are proportioned for your figure and have small prints or patterns. Wearing a single color has the effect of elongating your silhouette, while multiple colors tend to break up your shape, making you look smaller.

Short jackets, especially waist-length styles, will prevent you from appearing overwhelmed by your clothes. Knee-length, well-fitted skirts are good choice if you are not overweight. Figure-hugging pants will enhance your figure. Pants that end just above the ankle will also lengthen the legs. Baggy shirts and blouses can make you look dumpy; fitted tops and blouses are better.

Tips for women with large hips

Women with large hips should draw attention away from this area and accentuate the upper body instead. This can be achieved by using stronger colors and patterns on the top half and emphasizing the shoulders. Loose-fitting tops and long, loose-fitting jackets with wide lapels will make the hips appear narrower. Padded shoulders, puffed sleeves, wide-necked tops, scarves, and

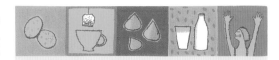

SUPER SHAPER

Black is an obvious choice when you are looking for clothes that will make you look slimmer; the "little black dress" has long been favored by women for just this reason. But while black can be slimming, it does not always flatter older women because it drains color from the face. Wearing the right colors can actually make you appear younger, enhancing your complexion and making your eyes sparkle. Stepping out in warm autumnal hues, pretty pastels, or bold, bright colors can lift your mood as well and will alter people's perception of you. One way to find out what suits you is to hold different colored fabrics up to your face and assess the impact. You can also enlist the help of an image consultant, who will judge which colors suit you by looking at the color of your eyes and hair and the tone of your skin.

shawls can all help to make the shoulders and neckline appear wider and thus balance the hips. Choose skirts with pastel or pale floral designs and wear them with darker colored or patterned tops.

Don't wear pleated skirts or styles that are too tight over the hips; these will make the hips look even bigger than they are. You should also avoid pattern details, motifs, and pockets placed at the hipline.

Tips for women with large busts

Large-busted women should aim to draw attention away from the upper body. Garments with a lower waistline make the bust seem more in proportion with the rest of the body. You can broaden and lengthen the appearance of the upper body by wearing long, loose-fitting jackets, tops, and tunics, especially styles with wide shoulders, shoulder pads, and V-necklines. It is best to avoid short sleeves, collars, and high necklines.

Wear long dresses with a belt set low on the hips and avoid skirts with wide waistbands. Avoid short tops and jackets, especially those with stripes, breast pockets, or fussy detail around the lapels.

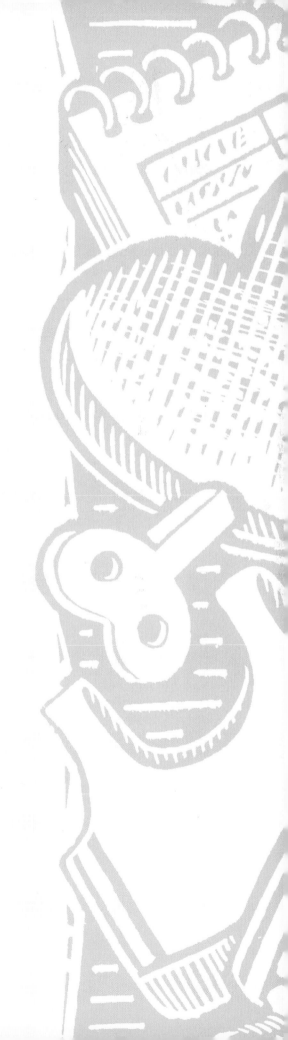

CHAPTER 4

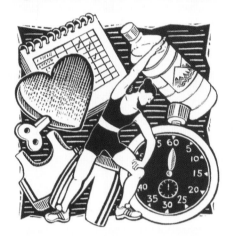

YOUR SHAPING-UP PROGRAM

A shaping-up program should be carefully planned. Setting exercise goals and knowing which exercises burn fat and which ones build muscle strength will help you tailor a regimen to your individual requirements. By understanding how muscles work and how best to improve their strength and flexibility, you can target specific areas to improve your shape and posture.

SETTING YOUR SHAPING-UP GOALS

The starting point for a shaping-up program is determining what you want to achieve, whether it's weight reduction, body toning, or strengthening of muscles.

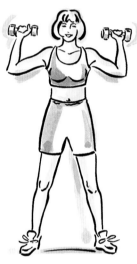

WHAT IS PROGRESSIVE RESISTANCE EXERCISE?
Progressive resistance training is defined as any muscular work that is performed against a resistance, such as a weight, with the aim of increasing muscular strength and tone. Typically, this resistance takes the form of free weights, such as barbells and dumbbells, or fixed weights, such as those found in gyms.

A shaping-up program should always be tailored to your goals. It is surprising how many people start an exercise regimen with no clear idea of what they want to achieve.

DECIDING ON YOUR GOALS

The human body has the capacity to transform itself in many different ways, depending on how it is challenged. Regular stretching of the muscles, for instance, can produce greater range of movement, while resistance training will lead to increased muscle tone. Before designing an exercise program, you should know what you are aiming for.

To decide if you need to lose weight, work out your BMI (see page 16). In order to achieve and maintain weight-loss goals, it is especially important to combine exercise with a controlled diet that is low in fat and high in complex carbohydrates and lean protein. You should also focus on aerobic forms of exercise, such as brisk walking, swimming, jogging, or cycling, which demand greater use of oxygen and are more efficient at burning fat (see page 83).

Aerobic exercise should also be the focus of your program if you want to improve your general level of fitness. Such exercise improves the functioning of your heart and lungs, the foundation of good general health. As your muscles are worked, they demand extra oxygen. The heart then pumps more oxygen-carrying blood around your body, improving its strength and efficiency over time.

When your weight and general fitness level are good, you can begin to focus your shaping-up program on muscle toning and strength building. If you want to improve the bulk of your muscles, you will need to perform high-resistance exercises, which involve lifting heavier weights over shorter periods of time. However, if you simply want to firm up your muscles without increasing bulk, you will have to do muscular endurance work. With this kind of exercise, resistance (the weight you are working against) is only moderate, and the emphasis is on working over longer periods of time.

Whatever your overall goals, joints must have a good range of movement for the body to move freely. You can achieve this through daily stretching of surrounding

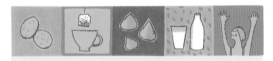

SUPER SHAPER

Swimming is a low-impact exercise that doesn't put strain on the body because it is supported by the buoyancy of the water. With each stroke, muscles are lengthened and strengthened (water is 12 times as resistant as air). Continuous swimming provides a good aerobic workout for the heart and lungs and can boost energy levels as well.

Aqua aerobics are a good alternative for people who don't enjoy swimming laps. They can be easier than normal aerobics classes yet yield the same effect because the exercises are done against the resistance of water. There are also water exercise classes specially designed for pregnant women. Because the buoyancy of the water prevents stress on joints, it is a safe way to exercise and tone the body, even late in a pregnancy.

DID YOU KNOW?

During exercise your heart rate speeds up to pump a greater volume of blood to the muscle groups being used. Depending on the type and intensity of the exercise, the amount of blood pumped around the body can increase from the usual 4 quarts a minute to as much as 27 quarts.

muscles. Healthy and attractive posture is dependent not only on sufficient muscular tone but also good flexibility. Your shape can improve dramatically simply as a result of holding yourself in better alignment and maintaining poised posture.

When setting your goals, try to make them realistic and attainable. Some people are born with body types best suited for endurance. The narrow shoulders and hips of long-distance runners, along with their naturally lean body composition, can never be transformed into the heavier, broad shape typical of power lifters.

The secret to success is making the most of what you have. Attempts to transform your body into something it was never meant to be will ultimately be fruitless and self-defeating.

CONSULT YOUR DOCTOR

Before starting your new exercise routine, it is a good idea to have a medical checkup, especially if you are older or unaccustomed to vigorous activity. Remember, however, that most general practitioners have no more knowledge of what various exercise programs involve than the average person, so it will be helpful if you give him or her a brief outline of what you intend to do and achieve. If you have sought advice from a fitness professional (see right), that person can compile a written description of the proposed activity, which you can then take along to show your doctor.

A medical checkup prior to exercise will focus mainly on identifying any existing risk factors for cardiovascular disease. You can expect to be asked about the health history of your biological parents and grandparents, your dietary habits, tobacco use, alcohol consumption, and stress levels. Your blood pressure will be taken and your heart listened to for any irregularities. Your cholesterol levels may also be tested. Be sure to discuss any other issues with your doctor that may affect the amount and kind of exercise you are able to do safely, such as arthritis, back problems, recent or old injuries, and joint or muscular concerns.

Getting advice

The better informed you become prior to undertaking a new exercise program, the safer and more effective it is likely to be. Seek advice from a qualified fitness expert. Employing the services of a personal trainer, at least in the initial stages of a new regimen, is strongly recommended. In addition, you can refer to the many fitness books and publications available at your local library.

WORKING EFFECTIVELY WITHIN SAFE LIMITS

Like other muscles, your heart can be trained to improve performance, but there are limits to what can be termed safe training. To stick within these limits, it is useful to determine your target training zone. Take your pulse 30 seconds after energetic exercise to check if you are working safely within your target zone. Over time, increase the intensity of your training but never work to your maximum heart rate (maximum heart rate equals 220 minus your age).

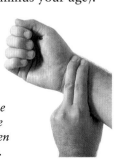

TAKING YOUR PULSE DURING TRAINING
Using two fingers, find your pulse on the inside of your wrist near your thumb. Because it will be slowing down, count the beats for 15 seconds, then multiply this count by 4.

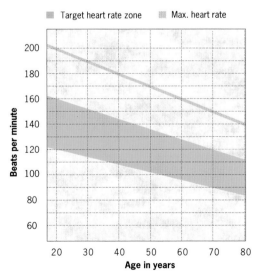

■ Target heart rate zone   ■ Max. heart rate

FINDING YOUR TRAINING ZONE
This graph shows the average target heart rates and maximum heart rates according to age. You should aim to exercise at between 65 and 85 percent of your maximum.

Best of both worlds
By combining resistance training with regular aerobic activity, you will improve your body shape as well as your overall fitness level. Aerobic exercise increases the efficiency of the heart, lungs, and circulatory system, whereas resistance work increases muscle strength and tone.

MONITORING YOUR PROGRESS

The establishment of long-term goals can be a powerful motivational tool, but breaking goals down into a series of progressive stages makes them less daunting and provides attainable short-term aims. Be realistic about the time span you allow for your achievements and be prepared to adapt your plan as necessary. Both long- and short-term goals need to be specific and measurable.

With regard to body weight, remember that the bathroom scale offers little insight into your fat/muscle ratio. A scale shows only your total body weight, which, due to fluid fluctuations, can vary from day to day. A better way to monitor your progress is to mix the factors being measured. Finding an improvement in your pulse rate taken at rest can be very encouraging because this will indicate an increase in your basic level of fitness. Recording your waist and hip measurements can be helpful as well, and keeping a diary in which you track your responses to your training regimen may provide an interesting record, hopefully revealing improvements in the amount of exercise that you can perform and the ease with which you can perform it.

HOW MUCH DO YOU NEED TO SHAPE UP?

The aim and course of your shaping-up program will be determined by your health and level of fitness at the outset.

This quiz can help you decide how much you need to shape up and on which areas your program should focus.

Do you get very breathless as a response to	When buying clothes, do you find getting a good fit	Do you suffer from aches and pains
(a) walking up stairs? (b) walking briskly? (c) jogging? (d) exercising hard?	(a) very difficult? (b) often a problem? (c) sometimes a problem? (d) no problem?	(a) constantly? (b) often? (c) occasionally? (d) rarely?
Do you smoke	Are your energy levels	Do you have difficulty in sleeping
(a) frequently? (b) socially? (c) seldom? (d) never?	(a) generally low? (b) fluctuating quite a lot? (c) okay most of the time? (d) generally high?	(a) a lot of the time? (b) sometimes? (c) once in a while? (d) rarely?
Is your BMI	Do you suffer from low spirits	Do you suffer from stiff joints
(a) obese? (b) overweight? (c) on the margin of overweight? (d) appropriate to your height?	(a) frequently? (b) occasionally? (c) sometimes, but it's manageable? (d) seldom?	(a) constantly? (b) frequently after exercise? (c) sometimes after intense exercise? (d) seldom?
Do you drink alcohol to excess	Do you exercise	Is your resting heart rate
(a) every day? (b) once a week? (c) once a month? (d) rarely?	(a) seldom? (b) occasionally? (c) once or twice a week? (d) more than twice a week?	(a) poor? (b) fair? (c) good? (d) excellent?

Mostly a's: You need to improve your general level of health with the guidance of your doctor. Your shaping-up program should focus on aerobic exercise to improve your cardiovascular health, but you should also look at other lifestyle factors, such as diet.

Mostly b's: Your general level of fitness could be improved with aerobic exercise. This will help you to control weight problems and may help you overcome any joint stiffness or low energy.

Mostly c's: Your general level of fitness is probably quite reasonable, but there are still areas in which you can improve. Your shaping-up program can focus more on toning your body and increasing your flexibility and strength to achieve a shape you're happy with.

Mostly d's: Your general level of fitness is very good. However, it is easy to let fitness slip. Your program should focus on muscle toning and maintaining your current activity levels.

THE IMPORTANCE OF STRETCHING

Whatever form of exercise you choose to undertake for your shaping-up program, proper stretching should be an integral part of it, both before and after exercise.

Healthy shape is not dependent only on good muscle tone; in order to hold good body alignment and posture, as well as to control movement, flexibility is essential, and for good flexibility you need to stretch your muscles regularly. Stretching is also essential in helping to avoid strain, and can prevent injury.

HOW MUSCLES STRETCH

Our skeletal muscles are generally attached to bones with tendons at each end of the muscle. When contracting, a muscle shortens and exerts a pulling force on the bones. As the two ends of the muscle draw toward each other, the bones move. In order for this to happen, the muscle must cross a joint.

Muscles can pull only; they cannot push. For this reason they always work in pairs, with their partner crossing the opposite side of the joint. For example, the biceps pull to flex the elbow, while at the same time, the triceps on the opposing side pull to extend it (see box, page 80). The range of movement around joints is therefore dependent not only on a muscle's ability to pull and create movement but also on its capacity to stretch and accommodate it. Flexibility training focuses on taking the two ends of any given muscle away from each other to challenge its ability to stretch.

HOW STRETCHING IMPROVES YOUR SHAPE

Posture describes the way in which bones are held up and carried by the skeletal muscles. When joints are correctly aligned, the nervous system and internal organs can function at optimal efficiency. Poor posture results in wasted energy and impedes the circulatory flow; the respiratory function decreases, and digestive problems may occur. Misaligned joints can lead to arthritis and chronic soft-tissue injuries, as well as lower back pain. You can transform your shape and appearance simply by improving your posture. A person carrying a few excess pounds of fat but holding it with poise and grace looks better than a slender individual who slouches; the good posture projects an image of self-confidence that is innately attractive.

DEVELOPMENTAL STRETCHING

Muscles have a built-in memory and automatically contract at their habitual limit. However, by holding a stretch until the muscle relaxes into the position, the limit can be extended. This new flexibility is then logged in the muscle's memory, increasing the muscle's capability. The exercise below stretches the muscles of the inner thigh.

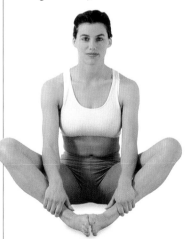

FIRST STAGE STRETCHING
Slowly ease your knees toward the floor. Hold for at least 10 seconds until you feel your muscles relax into the stretch.

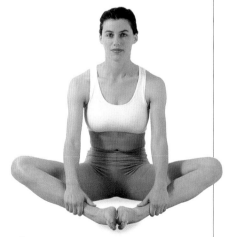

INCREASING THE STRETCH
Very slowly take the stretch further until you feel your muscles tensing once more. Hold for a minimum of 10 seconds.

The ability to achieve and maintain good posture depends on having both sufficient muscular tone and adequate flexibility. For example, the muscles of the upper back keep the shoulders from collapsing forward, but unless the chest can stretch to accommodate the position, rounded shoulders will result.

When flexed positions are consistently adopted, the muscles around the joints can become shortened and inflexible. This is known as adaptive shortening and is often seen in people who spend much of their daily lives sitting. When you are seated, both the hips and knees are flexed so that the hamstring muscles at the back of the thighs and the hip flexors at the front of the hip are in a shortened position. High-heeled shoes have a similar effect on calf muscles. The heel is unnaturally raised, resulting in bunching up of the muscles and their consequent loss of ability to extend.

Daily stretches for the muscles at the front of the chest and backs of the thighs and, especially for women, in the calf will help the body to become sufficiently elastic to accommodate a better posture.

THE STRETCH REFLEX

To prevent their becoming overextended, muscles have a self-protective mechanism that must be taken into account if stretching is to be safe and effective.

Every time the two ends of the muscle are taken to the limits of their range, a warning signal is transmitted to the brain via sensory nerves (see page 91). In response, the brain commands the muscle to contract to protect itself. This means that whenever you stretch, the initial result is actually a contraction. Only after the position has been held for a time and taken no further will the muscle relax. The time it takes for this reflex action to occur and then release is at least 6 seconds. Any stretch held for less than this amount of time is therefore ineffective.

METHODS OF STRETCHING

The most effective way to increase muscle elasticity is to perform developmental stretching, also known as proprioceptive muscular facilitation (PMF). You take the muscle to the limits of its range and hold it statically for 10 seconds or until you can

THE MECHANICS OF MUSCLE CONTRACTION

Skeletal muscles work in pairs to allow movement at a joint. As one muscle (the agonist) contracts, its opposite (the antagonist) must relax to allow the movement. If the antagonist is too short because of excessive tension or lack of exercise, for instance, movement will be restricted. A muscle that is too short will also impact on its opposite muscle, which can then become weak or overly stretched.

A muscle contains hundreds of elongated cells called muscle fibers (see page 87). Each fiber contains hundreds of myofibrils, and it is the shortening that occurs within these that causes the muscle itself to contract.

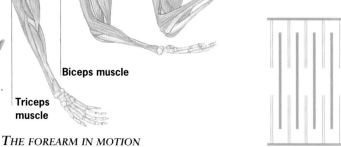

Biceps muscle

Triceps muscle

THE FOREARM IN MOTION
When the forearm is raised, the biceps bulks up and its opposite muscle, the triceps, stretches to allow movement. When the arm is lowered, the triceps contracts and the biceps relaxes.

THE SHORTENING OF THE MYOFIBRIL
In contraction the thick filaments contained in the myofibril slide in between the thin ones. It is this action that causes the muscle as a whole to contract.

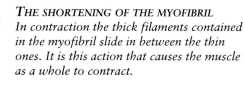

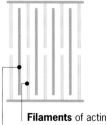

Filaments of actin
Thick strands of myosin

In a relaxed muscle
thick and thin filaments
overlap slightly.

In a contracted muscle
the thick strands slide in
between the thin ones.

CAUTION

Be careful about doing stretches if you have heart problems, high or low blood pressure, fever, sprain, strain, or inflammation or pain in joints. Relax a stretch if you feel the muscle trembling. Unless you are experienced, don't use a partner to help you do a stretch; you could force the muscle beyond the limits of its range.

feel the tension release. Once the stretch reflex has dispersed and the muscle has relaxed, it may be eased further. Initially it will contract again and must be given time to relax into its new position. You can repeat this gentle progressive lengthening two or three times for increased benefit. It is most effective in improving range of movement if performed daily.

Take care not to bounce, or pulse, when stretching as this continually triggers the stretch reflex and consequently leads to a buildup of tension within the muscle rather than the lengthening and relaxing needed to increase flexibility safely.

The more support the body has when stretching, the more relaxed it will be; therefore performing stretches on the floor, where appropriate, is particularly useful.

EFFECTIVE STRETCHING

When the partner of a muscle on the other side of a joint has to contract to bring about a stretch, this is known as an active stretch. For example, from a standing position, the heel of one leg can be pulled up toward the buttocks using the hamstrings on the back of the thigh. However, with so much tension in the back of the leg, it is very difficult for the quadriceps, which run down the front of the thigh, to relax into the stretch. A more effective stretch is achieved using the muscles of the arm to hold the leg in position. Then the entire thigh can relax. This method is known as passive stretching.

WHEN TO STRETCH

It is essential to lengthen your muscles prior to exercising in order to maximize their range of movement. Gentle stretching of the major muscle groups, such as the hamstrings at the back of the thigh and the adductors on the inner thigh, may also reduce the likelihood of injury. Pre-exercise stretches need to be held for a minimum of 10 seconds to be effective. Focus particularly on those muscles that will be involved in the activity you are about to do.

For developmental stretching to be safe and effective, muscles need to increase in pliability, which comes from warming them through movement. Attempting to stretch cold muscles may result in damage. Brisk walking, gentle cycling, even vigorous housework can all raise muscle temperature and enhance elasticity. Stretching is most efficient when the muscles are at their warmest, that is, after vigorous activity.

Stretching after exercise has been shown to be helpful in reducing muscle soreness, sometimes felt 24 to 48 hours after a tough workout. The relaxed lengthening of muscles and consequent reduction in their tension also has a calming effect on the mind and can help to ensure a sound night's sleep.

Before designing your stretch program, identify which joints feel adequately flexible and which ones feel restricted in their range of movement. For muscles that are already flexible, performing regular static stretches lasting 8 to 10 seconds will maintain their elasticity. For those muscles that are tight and limited in their range, performing daily developmental stretches will loosen them.

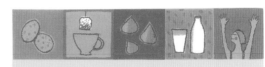

SUPER SHAPER

Jogging is an excellent way to warm up before a stretching session, and if you do it on a mini trampoline, you don't even have to leave the house. This inexpensive item of home equipment provides a means of ideal aerobic activity if you use it to your advantage; you can simply jog normally or you can bounce, lifting your arms up and down as you do so. Make sure the legs of the trampoline are secure and that there is enough head room for safe exercising. If you are a keen jogger, a trampoline means you are not limited to jogging during daylight hours and you do not have to go out when the weather is bad.

BALLISTIC STRETCHING

Ballistic stretching is the use of fast, jerky, or bouncing movements to increase a stretch. An example of this is bouncing to touch your toes. Ballistic stretches are sometimes used by professional gymnasts prior to specific actions but are generally not recommended for a number of reasons:

▶ *A fast stretch does not allow enough time for tissues to adapt and can lead to strain.*

▶ *A sudden jerk to a muscle will initiate the stretch reflex, and muscle tension will increase. Pulling against this tension can result in microscopic tears of the myofibrils. During healing, fibrous tissue will form, and it can impair muscle function.*

▶ *Bouncing movements are not easy to control. The positioning of joints and the direction of movement may not be correct, thus increasing the likelihood of injury.*

CASE STUDY

A Headache Sufferer

*The healthy functioning of your body is greatly affected by the way you hold yourself.
A sedentary lifestyle can result in muscles that are too weak and inflexible for good posture.
Poor diet and high stress levels compound the problem. By increasing muscle tone and
flexibility through exercise, you can improve your body's shape, health, and energy levels.*

Rita is a 31-year-old computer programmer who recently returned to work part-time following the birth of her second child. She has suffered digestive problems since college and during her pregnancy was diagnosed with irritable bowel syndrome (IBS), but since returning to work, she has started to feel run-down. She gets frequent headaches and has a stubborn respiratory infection, which she blames for her general aches and pains.

Rita knows her diet could be better; neither she nor her husband, Peter, are great cooks, and they eat a lot of packaged and take-out foods. She also feels she needs more exercise, but with young children, she has trouble finding the time.

WHAT SHOULD RITA DO?
Unhealthy eating and day-to-day stress are taking a toll on Rita's health. She needs a better diet—balanced, nutritious meals do not have to involve a lot of time or skill—and daily periods of exercise and relaxation. Some of her problems also stem from poor posture at work. She should have her computer positioned so that she can sit upright without tilting forward. Muscular toning and stretching exercises will improve her posture and, inevitably, her health. Doing simple, corrective exercises for two to three minutes every hour can strengthen the upper back muscles, realign the cervical vertebrae, and expand the chest, thus aiding the digestive system.

Action Plan

EMOTIONAL HEALTH
Set aside some time on a regular basis for relaxation, especially at the end of the day, which will promote sound sleep.

DIET
Eat more fresh fruits and vegetables every day. Start keeping a food diary to try to identify which foods spark the irritable bowel syndrome.

LIFESTYLE
Spend some time each day outdoors. Include exercise in the daily routine, even if it's just taking the children to the park.

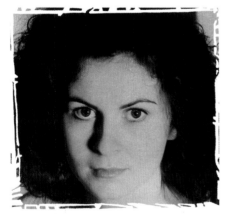

LIFESTYLE
Fresh air, natural light, and exercise are vital for both health and emotional well-being.

EMOTIONAL HEALTH
It is easy to forget your own needs when a family is making demands on your time and energy.

DIET
Too many processed foods can cause digestive distress. Caffeine and many condiments are also intestinal irritants. Wholesome fresh foods are the best choice.

HOW THINGS TURNED OUT FOR RITA

Rita had her computer raised to prevent her slouching. Now that she is aware of her posture, she does some stretches every hour. At home she makes an effort to get out with the children every day, and on weekends the whole family goes for a walk. She and Peter are both learning to cook and feel that their diet is much better. Rita has fewer headaches, the IBS is much improved, and she has far more energy than before.

THE PHYSIOLOGY OF FAT BURNING

If the main aim of your shaping-up program is to lose weight, it will undoubtedly help you to have an understanding of how fat is formed, stored, and utilized in the body.

The term *body fat* is used to describe a collection of thin-walled, oil-filled cells that lie mostly just beneath the skin. Each pound of fat stored in the body is the equivalent of 3,000 to 3,500 calories.

Fat is essential in our diet, helping to make available the valuable fat-soluble vitamins, A, D, E, and K, promoting healthy skin, and regulating body functions. However, most dietitians agree that the average Western person eats more fat than is required or is good for health. Excess fat that cannot be utilized as a fuel source by your body is stored as adipose tissue. Over time the excess can lead to problems with weight and to cardiovascular disorders.

Most people understand that exercise can help them utilize fat stores in the body, but exactly how does this occur?

HOW EXERCISE BURNS FAT

For muscles to contract, they must have a continual supply of phosphates, which the body provides by breaking down food. Carbohydrates are required in the greatest quantities because phosphates are most readily obtained from them. When consumed, carbohydrates are converted into glycogen, glucose, or fat. Glycogen is stored mainly in the liver and muscles, where it is available to provide phosphates for muscle

continued on page 86

BURNING FAT THROUGH DIET AND EXERCISE

In order to burn fat, exercise and diet must be modified. Studies show that the best way to burn fat is by performing low-intensity aerobic exercise for at least 20 minutes three times a week. Fat can be converted to energy only with the presence of oxygen. A short, intense burst of activity, such as a quick sprint, is anaerobic exercise, which means it does not use oxygen and it utilizes energy sources in the body other than fat. An hour's brisk walk, however, gets your cardiovascular system pumping oxygen to your muscles and mobilizes fat stores. Combined with a low-fat diet, this is the best way to burn fat.

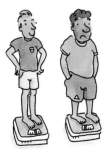

A healthy weight means you are eating the right amount of food for your activity levels. Overweight people eat more than they expend and so have excess stores of fat.

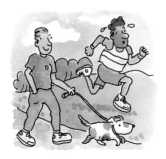

Regular low-intensity exercise, such as walking or cycling for an hour, will burn fat more effectively than short, intense bursts of exercise.

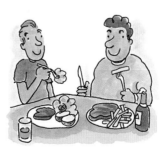

Following a low-fat diet will provide the right form of fuel for increased activity. High-fat food is less readily converted to energy by your body and so is stored as fat.

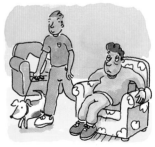

Your energy levels will be high as your body easily converts complex carbohydrates to fuel. With a high-fat diet you are more likely to feel fatigued by increased activity.

Very Overweight

The less fit you are, the harder exercising becomes. For people who carry a lot of excess weight, the challenge can seem daunting. But if the program is easy to perform, exercise can quickly become enjoyable—and produce results.

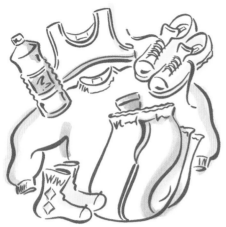

EQUIPPED FOR ACTION
Wear loose, comfortable clothing made of natural fibers, which absorb moisture, or of synthetic fibers that wick moisture away. Dress in layers so that clothing can be removed as you warm up. The ideal footwear is a pair of aerobic trainers. Always have a bottle of water at hand to make sure you don't become dehydrated.

Many heavily overweight individuals feel embarrassed to exercise in public, and so they try to lose weight by diet alone. This approach is unlikely to achieve the desired result; it often leads to yo-yo dieting and consequently a slower metabolic rate, which compounds the weight problem. Whatever your weight, the combination of a low-fat diet and well-planned, regular aerobic exercise is the quickest route to successful slimming and an increased feeling of well-being. Exercise will also boost your metabolism and firm up flabby areas so that your clothes will fit better even before you actually lose weight. Before you start to exercise, be sure you are dressed comfortably. For large-breasted women, a bra that provides good support is essential.

Excess body weight puts an unnatural pressure on the weight-bearing joints; to protect them when exercising, be sure to begin with flexibility exercises.

Always perform the movements slowly, aiming to achieve the biggest possible range of motion.

FLEXIBILITY EXERCISES

Most people reach peak flexibility around the age of 10. With advancing age, range of movement gradually decreases, and as muscles and tendons around joints shorten, stiffness occurs. This process often takes place more quickly in overweight people because they tend to do less exercise and their muscles become conditioned to less range of movement. The areas most commonly affected are the knees, lower back, hips, fingers, and toes. With regular stretching that takes your muscles beyond their normal range, you can slowly increase your flexibility and enjoy greater ease of movement.

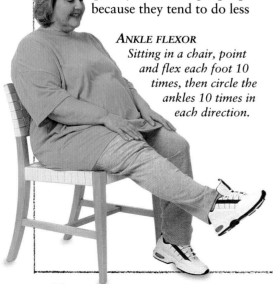

ANKLE FLEXOR
Sitting in a chair, point and flex each foot 10 times, then circle the ankles 10 times in each direction.

CIRCLING
Rotate each foot in a circle with a slow and controlled movement.

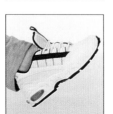

POINTING
Hold each point for 6 seconds. You will feel the stretch along the whole length of your lower leg.

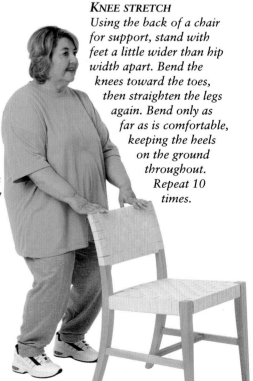

KNEE STRETCH
Using the back of a chair for support, stand with feet a little wider than hip width apart. Bend the knees toward the toes, then straighten the legs again. Bend only as far as is comfortable, keeping the heels on the ground throughout. Repeat 10 times.

AEROBIC EXERCISES

A common problem for greatly overweight people during exercise is skin burn. This occurs when one part of the body rubs against another while moving, resulting in chafing. Skin burn most commonly occurs on the inner thighs and underarms. The following exercises prevent skin burn while being effective aerobic conditioners. The number of times you repeat an aerobic exercise before moving on to the next can be increased as your fitness improves. Begin with 10 repetitions of each exercise and work up to 20. Once you can perform each exercise 20 times comfortably, aim to do the entire routine a second time. You may need to reduce the repetitions in the second run-through to 10 until your stamina improves. A good goal is eventually to be able to repeat the whole sequence 6 times through, performing each exercise 20 times.

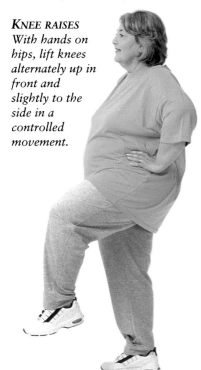

KNEE RAISES
With hands on hips, lift knees alternately up in front and slightly to the side in a controlled movement.

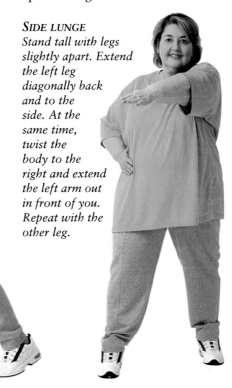

BACK LUNGE
Stand tall with legs slightly apart. Extend the left leg straight behind you, touching the ground with the ball of your foot only, while bending the right knee. As the leg goes back, extend your arms in front. Repeat with the other leg.

SIDE LUNGE
Stand tall with legs slightly apart. Extend the left leg diagonally back and to the side. At the same time, twist the body to the right and extend the left arm out in front of you. Repeat with the other leg.

WARMING UP AND COOLING DOWN

Start by performing some basic stretches for the back, legs, and shoulders (see Chapter 5). To allow your body to adapt gradually to the demands of the exercises, go through them slowly first without the arm work, then introduce the arms and increase the tempo as you feel more confident. Suddenly stopping after continuous activity can cause dizziness and contribute to the formation of varicose veins. To prevent this, finish each session by repeating the movements slowly, keeping the hands on the hips.

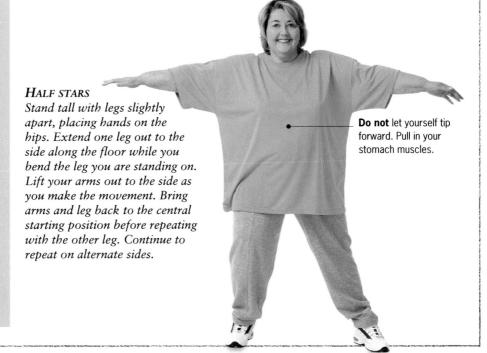

HALF STARS
Stand tall with legs slightly apart, placing hands on the hips. Extend one leg out to the side along the floor while you bend the leg you are standing on. Lift your arms out to the side as you make the movement. Bring arms and leg back to the central starting position before repeating with the other leg. Continue to repeat on alternate sides.

Do not let yourself tip forward. Pull in your stomach muscles.

contraction. Glucose circulates in the blood to feed the brain, kidneys, and red blood cells. Once glycogen and glucose stores are replenished, any extra carbohydrates are stored as fat, mostly under the skin and around the internal organs.

Although proteins are also a potential source of phosphates, their main role is to provide materials for cell building. Once the body's protein needs are met, any excess is converted to fat for storage.

Fat is a potential source of fuel, but in order for fat to be broken down for use, oxygen must be present. This means that most of the fat we eat is transferred directly into the fat stores of the body.

Many people believe that the intensity at which you perform exercise is the key to burning fat, but this is not necessarily the case. Aerobic exercise, which utilizes oxygen as the energy source, is the most effective at burning fat, and the longer it is performed, the more fat will be burned. If the intensity of the exercise causes you to become very out of breath, this is a sign that the oxygen supply is insufficient and therefore fat cannot be utilized. Forms of exercise such as weight lifting, sprinting, or ballet lifts, which involve sudden bursts of extreme activity, do not use the aerobic system. They use the anaerobic (without oxygen) system, which provides instant but unsustainable energy gained from glycogen rather than fat. Lactic acid may be produced as a by-product, and as levels build up, it creates a burning sensation in the muscles during exercise at high intensities.

CHECKLIST
There are several ways to monitor your progress during training.

✔ *Try the talk test (see below, left).*

✔ *Calculate your target training zone (see page 77) and check your pulse during training to make sure you stay within it.*

✔ *Take your resting pulse twice a week and keep a note of the count. A slower resting pulse indicates a fitness improvement.*

✔ *Use a scale of perceived exertion evaluated from 1 to 10, with 1 representing total inactivity and 10 maximum exertion. Effective fat burning for those unaccustomed to exercise takes place around 6 or 7 on the scale.*

✔ *Buy a heart rate monitor that straps around the chest and transmits the speed of cardiac contractions to a display worn on the wrist. An alarm will sound if you drop below or exceed your preset target heart rate.*

SPEEDING UP YOUR METABOLISM

While sustained exercise of lower intensity is the best way to utilize fat, exercise of higher intensity is more effective at raising your metabolic rate. This is the speed at which your body utilizes energy for all its basic functions. Exercise speeds up the resting metabolic rate (RMR) for some hours after exertion, meaning that more calories are burned up even when you are at rest.

The greater the intensity of exercise, the faster the metabolism speeds up and the longer it remains elevated. Research shows that it can remain higher for 24 hours or more after 30 minutes of vigorous activity.

Experts recommend at least 20 minutes of sustained aerobic exercise at least three times a week in order to achieve and maintain a moderate level of fitness. Obviously, the more exercise you do, the greater the fat-burning potential, but doing a little and often is considered more effective than sporadic, intense bursts. The aim should be to make aerobic exercise a regular feature of your daily life.

THE TALK TEST
Exercise increases your heart rate, making you breathe harder, but being greatly out of breath is a sign that you are overdoing it. It also means oxygen cannot be delivered to the muscle for fat burning, so your body is predominantly breaking down glycogen instead of fat for fuel. When exercising with a friend, monitor your breathing by holding a conversation. If you are exercising alone, attempt to sing or recite a rhyme.

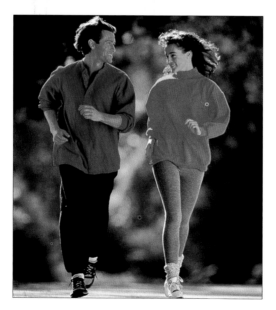

THE PHYSIOLOGY OF MUSCLE BUILDING

Understanding how muscles work can help you to plan an effective exercise program that will build up or strengthen muscles and prevent damage through excess or incorrect use.

The muscles of your body have four characteristics that set them apart from other types of tissue. These are excitability, that is, the capacity to receive and respond to nerve impulses; contractability, the power to contract; extensibility, the power to stretch; and elasticity, the capacity to return to their original shape. Any form of regular exercise that uses the muscles will therefore result in measurable changes in their tone and shape.

TYPES OF MUSCLE

There are three main types of muscle found in the body: heart, or cardiac, muscle, which has the capacity to beat at a constant steady rhythm without tiring; involuntary muscle, found, for example, in the gastrointestinal tract, which carries out other automatic functions; and voluntary, or skeletal, muscle, which is responsible for all conscious movement. It is the skeletal muscles, along with the skeleton and any stored fat, that determine your body shape.

Contractions by the skeletal muscles bring about movement or maintain posture. For example, when you walk along carrying a heavy load, the leg muscles are providing mobility, the arm muscles are supporting the load, and the muscles of the torso are keeping you upright. Skeletal muscles also produce a lot of heat energy—as much as 85 percent of body heat—which is the reason that exercise warms you up.

THE ANATOMY OF SKELETAL MUSCLE

It is the anatomy of skeletal muscles that enables them to contract. A muscle consists of dense groups of elongated cells called muscle fibers. These can be up to 1 foot long,

and they are held together in groups called fascicles by a sheath of connective tissue called the perimysium. Muscle fibers are fed with oxygen and glucose by the many capillaries that break through the perimysium. Within each muscle fiber are bundles of thinner fibers called myofibrils. These house

continued on page 90

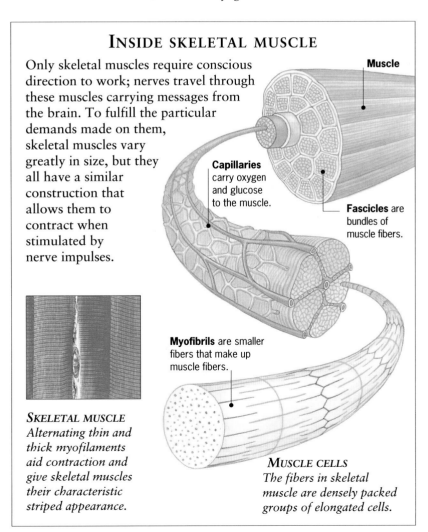

INSIDE SKELETAL MUSCLE

Only skeletal muscles require conscious direction to work; nerves travel through these muscles carrying messages from the brain. To fulfill the particular demands made on them, skeletal muscles vary greatly in size, but they all have a similar construction that allows them to contract when stimulated by nerve impulses.

Muscle

Capillaries carry oxygen and glucose to the muscle.

Fascicles are bundles of muscle fibers.

Myofibrils are smaller fibers that make up muscle fibers.

SKELETAL MUSCLE Alternating thin and thick myofilaments aid contraction and give skeletal muscles their characteristic striped appearance.

MUSCLE CELLS The fibers in skeletal muscle are densely packed groups of elongated cells.

Pilates Instructor

Favored by dancers for more than 70 years, Pilates is now gaining in mainstream popularity as a form of exercise that improves overall body tone and posture and increases flexibility without leaving you feeling exhausted.

A UNIVERSAL EXERCISE

Pilates first became popular with injured dancers, who used the system to regain strength and flexibility. In fact, Pilates can be beneficial for anyone, regardless of age and physical condition.

▶ *Pregnant women can use Pilates throughout pregnancy and after the birth to help regain their shape.*

▶ *The system can be adapted to suit any age or condition.*

▶ *Pilates not only tones every muscle but can also aid weight loss. Half an hour of Pilates exercises burns 180 to 220 calories.*

Pilates (pronounced pih-LAH-tees) is a system of exercise aimed at toning, stretching, and balancing the whole body. The movements are fluid and graceful, stretching out muscles to create sleekness rather than bulk. Instead of lifting weights or doing repetitions, practitioners focus on the quality of specific movements and stretches. Special equipment, unique to the Pilates method, is used in conjunction with exercises on the floor to achieve whole-body toning.

What are the origins of Pilates?

In the early 1900s German-born Josef Pilates, an athlete who was also asthmatic, studied both Eastern and Western exercise systems to develop his own personal bodybuilding program. During the First World War he worked as a nurse in England and experimented with attaching a system of springs to hospital beds to provide a way for patients to begin rehabilitation while still bedridden. The results were dramatic and led him to develop the Pilates system. He invented the Universal Reformer (see below) as part of this system, then went to America, where he started teaching his method; it quickly became popular with professional dancers, including the famous George Balanchine and Martha Graham.

What happens in a Pilates session?

Pilates training is usually done on a one-to-one basis, although some centers offer group classes for advanced students. Before you begin, the instructor will analyze your posture, looking at any areas of misalignment within the body. The session normally starts with a warmup and moves on to a series of

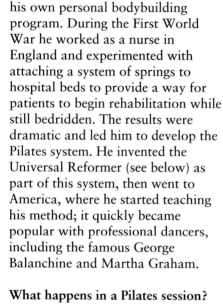

THE UNIVERSAL REFORMER
This contraption looks a bit like a torture rack, but the adjustable system of springs, straps, and bars can stretch all the muscles of the body using the person's own body weight as resistance.

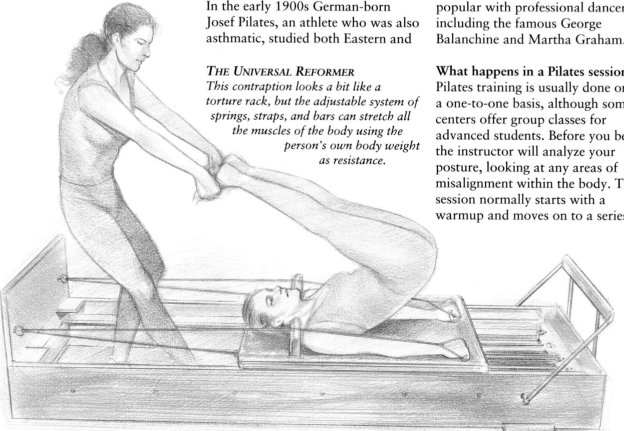

floor exercises designed to strengthen the center of the body—the muscles that circle the torso from the top of the hipbones to the base of the ribs. The floor work usually lasts for about 30 minutes. After this the session continues on the Universal Reformer, where every muscle of the legs can be worked, the back stretched, and the arms built up.

A beginner's program consists of a series of simple exercises that usually last for about 10 minutes (the time can extend up to 45 minutes for advanced students). The upper body is then exercised with the use of free weights and various other pieces of equipment. Individual postural requirements and physical needs are taken into consideration so that a tailor-made session, unique to the Pilates method, can be followed.

How fit do I need to be?

The Pilates method lends itself to all levels of physical fitness and all ages. Because classes are designed for each individual, Pilates can provide a tough workout for the fit and strong or a gentle stretching program for less able individuals.

Pilates is sometimes referred to as remedial gymnastics, and physio-therapists and doctors frequently prescribe it. This is because the technique can be worked around injured parts, giving the surrounding areas a thorough workout. It can also be used for rehabilitation to increase strength and flexibility once an injury has healed.

How quickly will I see results?

You will feel different—lighter, more balanced, and taller—after just one session. Many people report feeling energized, which sets the method apart from some workouts that can exhaust you. As with any exercise, regular practice is necessary to achieve the best results. Because it is a regimen that you can do at any age, there is no need to stop at any point. Many professional dancers and, in recent years, even football players have extended their careers by incorporating the method into their training.

What training do Pilates practitioners have?

Several Pilates studios in the United States can certify practitioners. Many students have already trained in another field, such as gymnastics, dance, or physiotherapy, before learning this system. Pilates training combines knowledge of exercise biomechanics and physiology with at least one year of rigorous practical training in the Pilates method. Some exercise instructors claim that their classes are Pilates based, but these are not true Pilates programs.

Can Pilates help with particular health problems?

The Pilates method can improve metabolism and benefit the nervous system. It can help ease migraines, tension headaches, depression, and seasonal affective disorder, and promote the health of the digestive, cardiovascular, and respiratory systems. It can also relieve some complaints of the musculoskeletal system, such as lumbar/sacral disc problems, knee pain, and pressure on cartilage or joints. The regular controlled exercise of the Pilates program can help as well to lower high blood pressure and relieve problems with the urogenital system, such as stress incontinence.

WHAT YOU CAN DO AT HOME

Once you are familiar with the Pilates way of moving and your body has improved in flexibility, there are a number of exercises you can practice at home in between Pilates sessions. These exercises usually concentrate on building strength in the abdominal region.

The exercise shown here, called the rolling ball, is performed in one slow and controlled continuous move-ment. If your abdominal muscles aren't strong enough to take you from the end of step 2 back to the starting position, you can build up some momentum by rocking gently back and forth. You will benefit most from the exercise if you perform it with 5 to 10 repetitions at least three times a week.

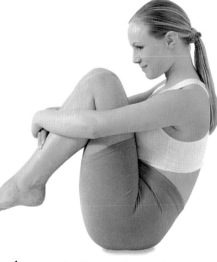

1 *Sit on the floor with your knees bent and pulled tightly into your chest. Wrap your arms around your legs with hands on your shins, then bring your nose toward your knees so that your spine is rounded slightly into a C shape. Lift your toes off the floor and balance on your buttocks.*

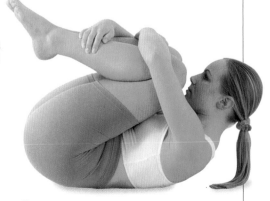

2 *Using your abdominal muscles, slowly roll backward to balance on your middle back and shoulder blades without altering the position of your arms and legs. In a continuous movement, roll forward to the starting position, keeping your heels as close as possible to your buttocks.*

even smaller filaments, actin and myosin, which are responsible for muscular contractions (see page 80). The actin and myosin filaments are divided up along the length of the muscle filament into sections called sarcomeres. Under a microscope, actin is seen as a thin line, while myosin is thicker and darker. The alternation of these two filaments gives skeletal muscle a distinctive striated, or striped, appearance.

When a muscle is stimulated to contract by a signal from the nervous system, the actin and myosin filaments draw toward each other like fingers being interlaced. This action causes the myofibrils, muscle fibers, and consequently, the overall muscle length to become shorter.

Connective tissue

Throughout the body there are various types of fibrous connective tissue, or fascia. In particular, fascia is found extensively within the muscles, where it reduces friction between a muscle's various components and also carries nerves, blood, and lymphatic vessels. Each muscle has three separate

DID YOU KNOW?

The human body contains more than 600 skeletal, or voluntary, muscles, all of which are constantly in contact with the brain. Each muscle is supplied with a nerve ending that transmits signals from the brain in a fraction of a second. However, messages that cause reflex actions, such as jerking away from a flame, do not travel all the way to and from the brain but use a self-preservation shortcut by interacting with the spinal column only. Thus, the speed of a reflex action is much faster than that of a conscious one, yet is completely beyond conscious control.

layers of fascia. These layers extend out from the ends of the muscles to form dense lengths of connective tissue called tendons, which mainly serve to attach muscles to bones. In some places the muscles are attached to other muscles by way of a broad, flat tendon known as an aponeurosis.

A characteristic that is common to all tendons is their relative lack of elasticity. They have far less potential to stretch than muscles and so are vulnerable to injury, especially when they are cold.

Ligaments, like tendons, are also made of dense connective tissue and are designed to give additional support to the joints. Ligaments are endowed with a limited degree of pliability in order to allow the joint to move, but they are positioned to prevent the joint from moving outside its intended range. If the ligaments were too elastic, the joints would be too unstable to permit controlled movement. Overstretched ligaments are a common cause of weak joints, especially in the ankles.

Connective tissue is greatly affected by temperature, becoming much more pliable when warm. A controlled program of gentle exercises and stretches that warm up the muscles and joints prior to vigorous exercise will reduce the likelihood of injury and enhance flexibility.

BUILDING MUSCLE

When muscles are regularly called on to cope with a heavier load than they have previously been used to, they respond to the extra demand by increasing the number of myofilaments inside the muscle cells. This

TENDONS AND LIGAMENTS OF THE HAND

Both ligaments and tendons are made up of dense fibers of connective tissue called collagen —a tough, flexible protein. The ligaments support bones, mainly in and around joints, to allow controlled movements and prevent a joint from overextending. Tendons provide a strong link between skeletal muscle and bone. Those in the hand extend up the arm to their controlling muscles situated near the elbow.

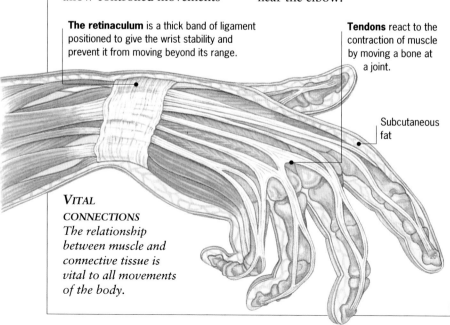

The retinaculum is a thick band of ligament positioned to give the wrist stability and prevent it from moving beyond its range.

Tendons react to the contraction of muscle by moving a bone at a joint.

Subcutaneous fat

VITAL CONNECTIONS The relationship between muscle and connective tissue is vital to all movements of the body.

HOW MUSCLES GUARD AGAINST DAMAGE

The brain sends commands to the muscles via the motor nerves of the central nervous system. The initial effects of resistance training mainly occur within these nerve pathways as the body learns to stimulate muscle fibers in the correct sequence to accomplish the movement. Muscles guard against damage by automatically reducing their work output or stopping in the face of fatigue. This is called the principle of inhibition.

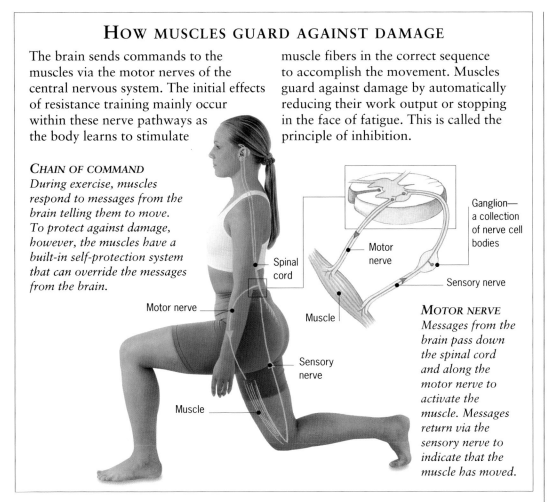

CHAIN OF COMMAND
During exercise, muscles respond to messages from the brain telling them to move. To protect against damage, however, the muscles have a built-in self-protection system that can override the messages from the brain.

Ganglion—
a collection
of nerve cell
bodies

Motor
nerve

Spinal
cord

Sensory nerve

Motor nerve

Muscle

Sensory
nerve

Muscle

MOTOR NERVE
Messages from the brain pass down the spinal cord and along the motor nerve to activate the muscle. Messages return via the sensory nerve to indicate that the muscle has moved.

causes an increase in the size of the muscle fibers, a process known as hypertrophy, thus strengthening them.

The way that muscles respond to different forms of exercise is determined by the type of fiber being used. Muscles contain three types of fiber: slow-twitch, fast-twitch, and intermediate-twitch. Slow-twitch fibers are thin and have a plentiful supply of capillary blood vessels. They also contain a large store of myoglobin, which increases their oxygen supply, and numerous mitochondria (see page 59), structures in which aerobic energy production occurs. Their primary source of fuel is fat, which, along with their rich oxygen supply, gives them a high endurance level. This means they can carry out low-intensity tasks for long periods of time, provided that oxygen can be supplied to meet their needs. However, their narrow size limits their power and intensity.

Fast-twitch fibers are double the width of slow-twitch fibers. They have large reserves of glycogen but are poorly supplied with blood capillaries and mitochondria, so they are powered by anaerobic energy systems. Because of their large size, they can contract in a sudden, powerful way to overcome high resistance, requiring no oxygen to do so. But they lack endurance and tire quickly.

Intermediate-twitch fibers, which are between the other two types in size, are more powerful than slow-twitch fibers. They are well supplied with capillaries and mitochondria and thus are powered by the aerobic system, giving them some endurance but not as much as that of slow-twitch fibers.

All muscles contain a mixture of these types of fiber but in varying proportions, depending on the muscle's function. Partly for genetic reasons but also in response to training, some people have more of particular fiber types than others. The leg muscles of marathon runners, for example, consist of about 80 percent slow- and intermediate-twitch fibers, whereas sprinters' leg muscles contain about 60 percent fast-twitch fibers. The legs of weight lifters are made up of an equal mixture of both fast- and slow/intermediate-twitch fibers.

MUSCLE INTELLIGENCE
During training, a long-distance runner focuses on muscular endurance and long-term energy release from muscles. The muscles respond to regular training by increasing the percentage of slow-twitch fibers, which have a high endurance level. If the person were to give up long-distance running and take up sprinting, the muscles would respond by increasing in fast-twitch fibers, which are more powerful for high-intensity work.

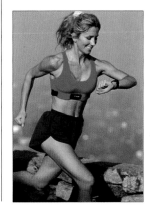

An exercise overview
The American College of Sports Medicine recommends that for health benefits people should do resistance training twice a week. They suggest that each session take a whole-body approach, including 8 to 12 exercises for the major muscle groups. It is not only muscles that become stronger with strength training but also tendons, ligaments, and bones.

Slow-twitch and intermediate-twitch fibers respond to training by improving their ability to utilize oxygen. Regular endurance training increases the number of capillaries, which enhances the body's ability to transport carbon dioxide and oxygen. The mitochondria also increase in number and size. The overall effect is enhanced muscle tone. Fast-twitch fibers have the potential to bulk up with high-intensity resistance training.

Whether an exercise program will increase muscle size or simply enhance muscle tone depends on whether training focuses on resistance work or endurance.

Regular exercise makes the muscle fibers more efficient, so fewer muscle fibers are needed for any given strength exercise. This leaves others free to take over when some become exhausted. Such economy of effort means that work can be continued for a longer time, producing endurance benefits.

Building and toning
The term *muscle building* suggests the development of greater muscle mass, and it is possible to design a training program that will result in larger muscles. But it is also possible to become stronger and to improve endurance without substantially increasing the size of muscles.

Many women avoid strength training because they worry about developing a masculine-looking body. But unless a woman is born with an above average number of fast-twitch fibers and abnormal levels of the male hormone testosterone, which aids muscle building, and then trains diligently at high intensities, she is unlikely to produce abnormal muscle bulk.

Because the body responds in very specific ways according to how it is challenged, a program of resistance training can be designed to achieve either muscular bulk or simply a heightened state of tone.

To bring about improvements in muscle strength or endurance, muscles must be regularly challenged to work at a level just beyond their present capabilities. This is known as applying overload. To increase in strength, the muscle must overcome progressively greater resistance, whereas to improve in endurance, it must perform the exercise for a gradually extended period. The ways in which muscles adapt in response to overload are called the training effects.

Improving muscle tone without increasing bulk
To improve muscle tone without significantly increasing muscle bulk, you should focus on challenging the slow-twitch fibers. You can do this by working with levels of resistance that are moderate enough to allow many repetitions.

Because of the low endurance capabilities of fast-twitch fibers, developing strength involves a few repetitions repeated several times in groups, or sets, with rest or recovery periods inserted between each set. In comparison, endurance training focuses on the slow and intermediate fibers and thus requires lower levels of resistance. It involves fewer sets but a higher number of consecutive repetitions, thereby challenging the stamina of muscles. When designing your own program for improving your shape, remember the benefits of strength work as well as endurance training.

EVERYDAY MUSCLE USAGE

Many of our muscles get used at some point during the day; a few examples are listed below. Because of increasingly sedentary lives, however, many muscles are underworked. When a sedentary person performs an out-of-the-ordinary task, such as mowing the lawn, underworked muscles can become quickly fatigued.

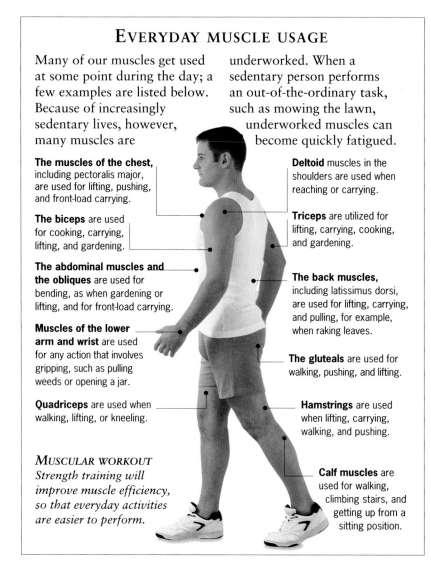

The muscles of the chest, including pectoralis major, are used for lifting, pushing, and front-load carrying.

The biceps are used for cooking, carrying, lifting, and gardening.

The abdominal muscles and the obliques are used for bending, as when gardening or lifting, and for front-load carrying.

Muscles of the lower arm and wrist are used for any action that involves gripping, such as pulling weeds or opening a jar.

Quadriceps are used when walking, lifting, or kneeling.

MUSCULAR WORKOUT
Strength training will improve muscle efficiency, so that everyday activities are easier to perform.

Deltoid muscles in the shoulders are used when reaching or carrying.

Triceps are utilized for lifting, carrying, cooking, and gardening.

The back muscles, including latissimus dorsi, are used for lifting, carrying, and pulling, for example, when raking leaves.

The gluteals are used for walking, pushing, and lifting.

Hamstrings are used when lifting, carrying, walking, and pushing.

Calf muscles are used for walking, climbing stairs, and getting up from a sitting position.

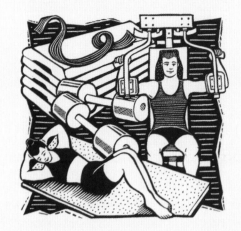

EXERCISES TO SHAPE UP YOUR BODY

This chapter provides step-by-step photographs and instructions for exercises to strengthen and shape up your whole body. Each exercise is safe for most people to perform, from beginners to the more advanced. Tables at the beginning of the chapter provide a guide to the number of times each exercise should be done, according to the level of fitness.

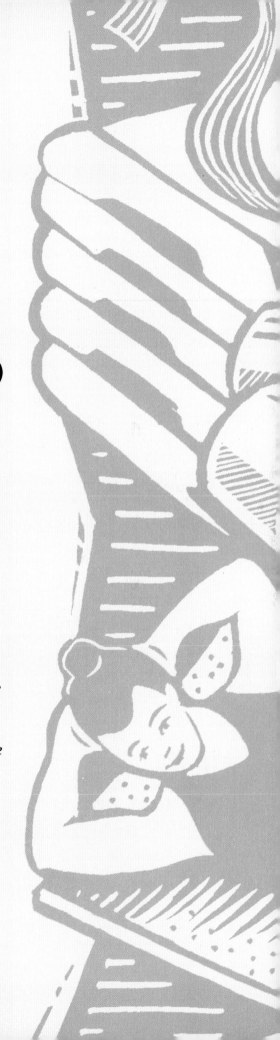

BEGINNING TO EXERCISE

Embarking on an exercise program can lead the way to a much better shape. On the following pages you will find exercises designed to develop strength, muscle tone, and flexibility.

Whether you want to be in better condition to play a sport or just want to gain all-round improvement in your strength and shape, you need to know how the different muscle groups work and the best way to tone and strengthen them. If you wish to improve a particular part of your body because it is weak from an injury or lack of use, or if you want to strengthen your body overall in order to perform a particular task, you will find a number of different exercises in this chapter to help you achieve your goal.

HOW TO USE THIS CHAPTER

The exercises that appear on the following pages are organized according to the muscle groups of the body, beginning with the head and neck. Most of the movements can easily be performed at home with no special equipment. However, some useful exercises that require the machines found in gyms have also been included.

To shape up your whole body, work through the entire chapter, performing each set of exercises methodically. They are designed for both men and women. Although people often desire different results from an exercise program—men may seek to look and feel stronger, whereas women usually want to become firmer and slimmer—the means of achieving these goals are much the same.

The charts on pages 96 and 97 provide a general guide to the number of times you should do each exercise depending on the condition of your body; it's important to know what your basic fitness level is before starting any kind of exercise program. Also, before doing any of the exercises shown, you must warm up thoroughly. This is of particular importance if you are stretching your muscles or using any kind of weights. If you do not warm up first, you could tear a muscle or incur another type of painful and debilitating injury.

A good warmup is to walk or jog in place for at least five minutes. While you are walking, swing your arms to loosen your joints. Begin your warmup slowly, gradually increasing the level of exertion as you continue; this will help you avoid much of the stiffness that many people experience the day after exercising.

Each section of this chapter begins with an illustration of the principal muscles in the part of the body being addressed and a description of some common shape problems in this area. Basic stretches precede

RESISTANCE EQUIPMENT

Although you can perform most exercises effectively without any special equipment, in some instances—particularly if you are at an intermediate or advanced level—dumbbells, wrist and ankle weights, and an elastic band may be very helpful. You can wear wrist and ankle weights while performing more active forms of exercise to provide a greater challenge or use elastic bands and dumbbells to develop greater strength and tone during controlled exercises. Any of these items are available at a sporting goods store or can be used free of charge at a health club.

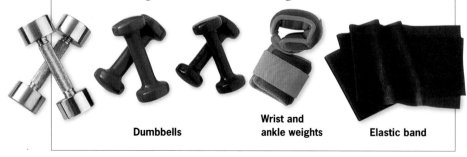

Dumbbells **Wrist and ankle weights** **Elastic band**

each group of exercises. It is important to perform these first to allow your muscles to get used to the movement before you begin toning in earnest. It is also essential to cool down after exercising, especially if you have pushed yourself hard. Relax by doing some gentle stretches, then treat yourself to a soothing aromatherapy bath.

Each muscle in the body works as part of a pair (see page 80). This is why you should complete the whole sequence of an exercise to ensure that each partner within the pair is strengthened equally. If one muscle becomes stronger through a great deal of use, its companion muscle could become weaker and shortened and ultimately cause posture problems and pain. You should also try to make sure that your body is strengthened all over. If you have one area that is weak, others may have to compensate for it and you could find yourself in pain.

If you suffer from any medical condition, such as heart disease or diabetes, or if you are pregnant, you should consult your doctor before you begin exercising. There may be certain exercises that you should avoid or others that could be particularly beneficial to your health.

THE MAIN MUSCLES OF THE BODY

There are more than 600 muscles in the human body; each one works as part of a pair to allow the body sufficient strength and flexibility to carry out everyday activities. Skeletal muscles are attached to bones and cross joints, providing them with the force to move. Muscles are layered in the body and often overlap each other. Those that are located just below the skin are known as superficial muscles; lying beneath them are the deep muscles. Your goal should be to use all of your muscles regularly so that none become atrophied. The larger muscles and the ones most commonly targeted in exercise programs are shown here.

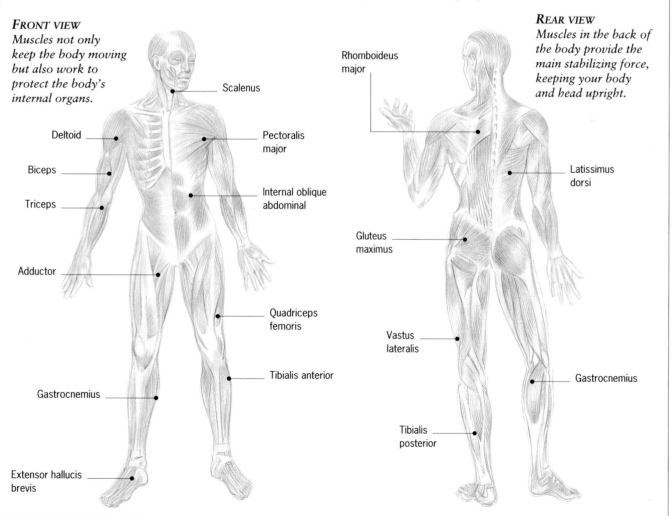

FRONT VIEW
Muscles not only keep the body moving but also work to protect the body's internal organs.

Scalenus

Deltoid

Pectoralis major

Biceps

Triceps

Internal oblique abdominal

Adductor

Quadriceps femoris

Tibialis anterior

Gastrocnemius

Extensor hallucis brevis

REAR VIEW
Muscles in the back of the body provide the main stabilizing force, keeping your body and head upright.

Rhomboideus major

Latissimus dorsi

Gluteus maximus

Vastus lateralis

Gastrocnemius

Tibialis posterior

A General Exercise Program

*One of the most important aspects of an exercise program is establishing
clear and realistic short- and long-term goals that will help you maintain motivation
and measure improvements. The four programs on these two pages provide a general guide for
building strength, tone, and mobility for every level of fitness over a 12-week period.*

To select the right exercise program, you should first take your resting pulse rate (see page 86), which will give you a general idea of your basic level of fitness. Each program works all the main muscle groups and should be followed in the order shown in the chart. The word *reps* refers to the number of times to perform a movement; *set* is the total number of repetitions. You should allow a 30-second rest between each set. Follow the program at least twice a week and always include a warmup and cooldown period and stretches before and afterward.

BEGINNER'S PROGRAM

		WEEKS 1–4			WEEKS 5–8			WEEKS 9–2		
BODY PART	EXERCISE	SETS	REPS	WEIGHT	SETS	REPS	WEIGHT	SETS	REPS	WEIGHT
Chest	Push-up (easy)	1	10–20	-	2	10–20	-	3	10–20	-
Back	Seated row with band	1	10–20	-	2	10–20	-	3	10–20	
	Superman	1	10–20	-	2	10–20	-	3	10–20	-
Shoulders	Dumbbell lateral raise	1	10–20	-	2	10–20	-	3	10–20	-
Legs	Squat	1	10–20	-	2	10–20	-	3	10–20	-
	Inner thigh raise	1	10-20	-	2	10–20	-	3	10–20	-
	Outer thigh raise	1	10–20	-	2	10–20	-	3	10–20	-
Abdominal	Basic crunch	1	10–20	-	2	10–20	-	3	10–20	-
muscles	Oblique curl	1	10–20	-	2	10–20	-	3	10–20	-

INTERMEDIATE PROGRAM

		WEEKS 1–4			WEEKS 5–8			WEEKS 9–12		
BODY PART	EXERCISE	SETS	REPS	WEIGHT	SETS	REPS	WEIGHT	SETS	REPS	WEIGHT
Chest	Push-up (easy)	2	10–20	-	3	10–20	-	3	10–20	-
	Flat bench or incline fly	1	10–20	-	2	10–20	-	3	10–20	-
Back	Seated row with band	2	10–20	-	3	10–20	-	3	10–20	-
	Superman	2	10–20	-	2	10–20	-	3	10–20	-
	Reverse fly	1	10–20	-	2	10–20	-	3	10–20	-
Shoulders and	Dumbbell lateral raise	2	10–20	-	3	10–20	-	3	10–20	-
arms	Triceps dip	1	10–20	-	2	10–20	-	3	10–20	-
	Biceps curl	1	10–20	-	2	10–20	-	3	10–20	
Legs	Squat	3	10–20	-	3	10–20	-	3	10–0	-
	Inner thigh raise	2	10–20	-	3	10–20	-	3	10–20	-
	Outer thigh raise	2	10–20	-	3	10–20	-	3	10–20	-
	Glute lift	1	10–20	-	2	10–20	-	3	10–20	-
Abdominal	Prone extension stretch	2	10–20	-	3	10–20	-	3	10–20	-
muscles	Basic crunch	2	10–20	-	3	10–20	-	3	10–20	-
	Ab trainer crunch	1	10–20	-	2	10–20	-	3	10–20	-
	Oblique curl	1	10–20	-	2	10–20	-	3	10–20	-

ADVANCED PROGRAM

BODY PART	EXERCISE	WEEKS 1–4			WEEKS 5–8			WEEKS 9–12		
		SETS	REPS	WEIGHT	SETS	REPS	WEIGHT	SETS	REPS	WEIGHT
Chest	Push-up (advanced)	3	10–20	-	3	10–20	-	3	10–20	-
	Flat bench or incline fly	2	10–20	-	3	10–20	-	3	10–20	-
	Flat dumbbell press	1	10–20	-	2	10–20	-	3	10–20	-
Back	Seated row with band	3	10–20	-	3	10–20	-	3	10–20	-
	Superman	3	10–20	-	3	10–20	-	3	10–20	-
	Reverse fly	2	10–20	-	3	10–20	-	3	10–20	-
	Single arm dumbbell row	1	10–20	-	2	10–20	-	3	10–20	-
Shoulders and arms	Dumbbell shoulder press	1	10–20	-	2	10–20	-	3	10–20	-
	Dumbbell lateral raise	2	10–20	-	3	10–20	-	3	10–20	-
	Triceps dip	3	10–20	-	3	10–20	-	3	10–20	-
	Biceps curl	3	10–20	-	3	10–20	-	3	10–20	-
Legs	Squat	2	10–20	-	3	10–20	-	3	10–20	-
	Lunge—single leg	1	10–20	-	2	10–20	-	3	10–20	-
	Inner thigh raise	3	10–20	-	3	10–20	-	3	10–20	-
	Outer thigh raise	3	10–20	-	3	10–20	-	3	10–20	-
	Glute lift	3	10–20	-	3	10–20	-	3	10–20	-
Abdominal muscles	Prone extension stretch	3	10–20	-	3	10–20	-	3	10–20	-
	Basic crunch (advanced)	2	10–20	-	3	10–20	-	3	10–20	-
	Ab trainer crunch	2	10–20	-	3	10–20	-	3	10–20	-
	Oblique curl (advanced)	2	10–20	-	2	10–20	-	3	10–20	-

GENERAL MOBILITY PROGRAM

Many people neglect their flexibility when developing an exercise program, but good flexibility is vital for overall mobility and ease of movement. As you age, especially if your occupation is primarily sedentary, you may find that your muscles have become weaker and shortened. This can lead to stiffness and aches that can seriously limit your general level of activity and ability. Doing the exercises below regularly should help you maintain good strength and suppleness. One caution, if you suffer from arthritis or any other serious joint or bone disorder, you should discuss your exercise plans with your doctor first.

BODY PART	EXERCISE	WEEKS 1–4			WEEKS 5–8			WEEKS 9–12		
		SETS	REPS	WEIGHT	SETS	REPS	WEIGHT	SETS	REPS	WEIGHT
Neck	Head rotation	1	10	-	2	10	-	3	10	-
	Deep neck extensor	1	10–20	-	2	10–20	-	3	10–20	-
	Upper trapezius stretch	-	1			2		-	3	-
	Scalene stretch	-	1			2		-	3	-
Hands	Wrist mobility exercises	1	10–20	-	2	10–20	-	3	10–20	-
	Wrist strengthening—ball	1	10–20	-	2	10–20	-	3	10–20	-
	Wrist extensor stretch	-	1		-	2		-	3	
	Wrist flexor stretch	-	1		-	2		-	3	
Feet	Arch exercise	1	10–20	-	2	10–20	-	3	10–20	-
	Dorsi flexion	1	10–20	-	2	10–20	-	3	10–20	-
	Toe extensors stretch	-	1		-	2		-	3	

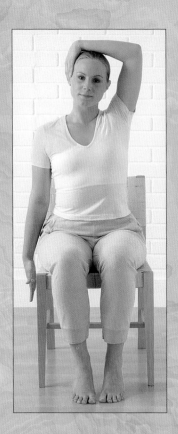

Head and Neck

The muscles of the head and neck are often neglected in exercise routines. Exercising and stretching these muscles regularly can help to prevent muscular pain, stiffness, fatigue, and headaches.

The muscles of the face usually get enough exercise from the range of normal facial expressions to maintain adequate tone. However, an important group of muscles that move the head and cervical spine do require regular toning exercise.

The sternomastoids, two prominent and powerful muscles at the front and sides of the neck, are attached to the top of the breastbone and the collarbone and connected to the skull just below the ear. Their main actions are to pull the head to the side (lateral flexion) and rotate the head in the opposite direction. Both sternomastoids work together to lift the head from a prone position and to help lift the chest during heavy exertion. In adults the head

weighs about 11 pounds, so the sternomastoids need to be fairly strong. Either of these muscles can be felt easily; place your left index finger on the end of your left collarbone (in the hollow of the throat). Now turn your head slowly to your right and you will feel the sternomastoid muscle push against your finger as it contracts.

The scalenes, triangular muscles that are joined to the front of the neck (cervical) vertebrae and the first rib, can bend the neck forward (flexion) and to the side (lateral flexion) and rotate the head to the opposite side. The scalenes also aid respiration during heavy exertion by lifting the first rib, thus allowing more space for the lungs to expand.

COMPLEMENTARY EXERCISES FOR THE NECK

▶ Yoga is an excellent form of exercise for the neck muscles. Many yoga postures extensively stretch and strengthen them.

▶ Swimming is a safe way in which to extend the neck muscles through a range of movements because water supports the weight of the head while you swim.

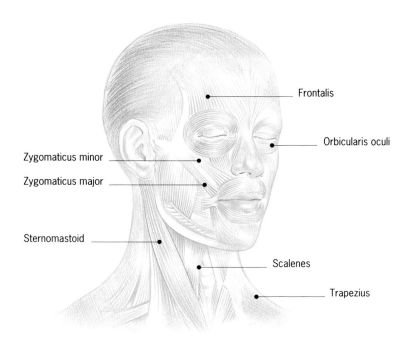

Frontalis

Orbicularis oculi

Zygomaticus minor

Zygomaticus major

Sternomastoid

Scalenes

Trapezius

Exercises to target the neck

Performing stretching exercises to increase flexibility and strength in the neck and facial muscles can make a difference to the rest of your workout. The upper body in many people is very stiff and tense, causing headaches and excessive tiredness at the end of the day. Increasing the suppleness of your neck muscles can greatly improve your energy levels.

NECK STRETCHES

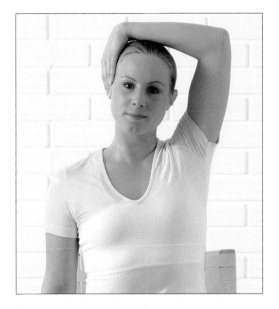

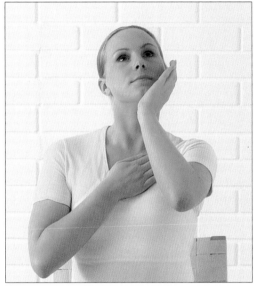

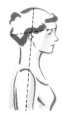

Don't allow your lower back to overarch. This places stress on the vertebrae of the lower back and may cause pain.

Don't let your head fall backward. This places stress on the vertebrae at the back of the neck.

Upper trapezius stretch
Sit on a chair with back upright and shoulders level. Pull your right hand slightly toward the floor with fingers pointing down. Place your left hand over the right ear and ease your head slightly to the left until you feel a mild stretch. Hold for 10 to 30 seconds, breathing evenly. Slowly release and repeat on the other side.

Scalene stretch
Sit on a chair with your back straight. With your left hand, support your chin in a slightly raised position. Rest your right hand on your sternum and rotate your head slightly to the right. Look up and depress the sternum with your right hand until you feel a mild stretch. Hold for 10 to 30 seconds. Release and repeat on the other side.

Head rotation
This exercise stretches the sternomastoids and scalenes. Sit upright in a chair. Slowly turn your head to one side, stopping as soon as you feel a mild stretch. Hold for 10 seconds; return to the starting position and stretch the other side. Repeat 5 to 10 times.

Deep neck extensors
While doing this exercise, you should sit in a chair that has a rigid, low back.

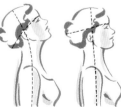

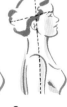

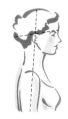

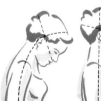

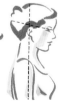

1. Begin by tilting your head back slightly.

2. Draw your chin forward and level your head.

3. Keeping your head level, return to the upright position.

4. Tilt your chin toward your chest.

5. Ease your head backward, keeping your chin down.

6. Slowly raise chin and head back to upright position.

The Chest

The shape of your chest can be determined by many factors: your body type, your diet, the amount and type of exercise you perform, and your habitual posture. There is much you can do to improve its shape with specific strengthening exercises.

The chest muscles can be a source of shape problems for both men and women. Typically, men are often concerned about weak chest muscles or a sunken appearance, while many women worry about their breast shape. Strong chest muscles are important for everyone; we all need a certain amount of strength for the tasks of lifting and carrying. Strong chest muscles also support good posture, which in turn prevents aches and pains and improves the efficiency of the lungs.

The anatomy of the chest
The large pectoral muscle, or pectoralis major, is the biggest and most powerful muscle of the chest. This triangular muscle is joined to the upper torso in two places: a small portion is connected to the collarbone, or clavicle, while the larger part is linked to the breast bone, or sternum. All the fibers of the muscle converge into a flat tendon that is attached to the upper arm bone. In women, a large portion of the breast overlies the

COMPLEMENTARY EXERCISES FOR THE CHEST

▶ Swimming, especially the breaststroke, crawl, and butterfly, promotes strong pectorals.

▶ The reaching shots in racquet sports require and enhance strong pectorals.

▶ Posture can make a huge difference to your chest shape. The Alexander technique (see pages 47–48) can help you improve rounded shoulders or a weak back.

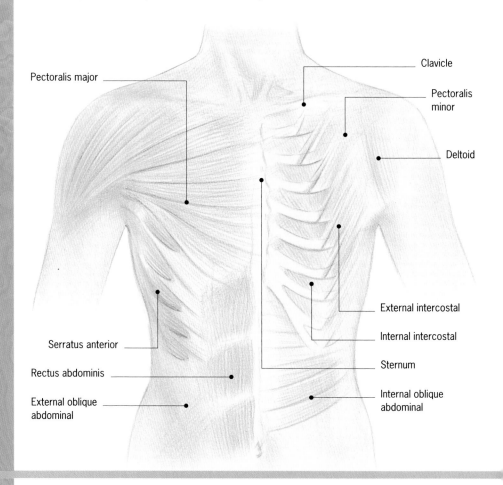

Pectoralis major

Clavicle

Pectoralis minor

Deltoid

External intercostal

Internal intercostal

Serratus anterior

Rectus abdominis

Sternum

External oblique abdominal

Internal oblique abdominal

pectoralis major. The main action of this muscle is to draw the arm across the front of the body, a movement known as adduction. The whole of the muscle can be made to contract by placing the hands together in front of the body and pressing them together.

The pectoralis major consists of two main parts that often work independently and so are sometimes referred to as the upper and lower pectoral muscles. During heavy exertion the whole muscle may also be used to aid breathing.

Another muscle, the deltoid, works along with the pectoralis major to perform many movements. But its principal role is to lift the arm forward from the side of the body, an action called flexion.

Underneath the pectoral muscle is a smaller triangular muscle called the pectoralis minor. This is linked to the third, fourth, and fifth ribs and the shoulder blade. It moves the shoulder blade forward and down and also acts as a stabilizer.

Chest problems

When the chest muscles weaken with lack of use, the result is sagging pectorals in a man. Certain strengthening exercises can tone the pectorals and over time restore their firmness, but it is important to consider diet as well as exercise. Cutting back on high-fat foods will do much to improve the shape of the chest.

Breast problems

The breasts lie over the muscles of the chest and are mainly composed of fat; therefore, exercises aimed at changing breast size usually have limited success. When a woman has large breasts and excess body fat, a program designed to reduce overall body fat levels will generally lead to a reduction in breast size too. All women, however, can benefit from exercises to tone the pectoral muscles that underlie the breasts.

SHAPE CHALLENGE
Sagging breasts

Many women experience a loss of breast firmness as they age or after breast-feeding. Unfortunately, because of the anatomy of the breast, a sagging bustline can be difficult to overcome. The firmness of the breasts is dependent on the suspensory ligaments (see page 71). These ligaments are nonelastic and, once stretched, for instance, by significant weight gain, cannot be restored to their original size. However, exercise can do much to improve breast shape by strengthening the chest muscle that lies below the breast.

CASE HISTORY

Suzy is a 37-year-old woman with a 12-month-old son, Paul. Since weaning Paul six months ago, she has been trying to restore her breasts to their former shape but has had little success. Suzy has begun attending aerobics classes twice a week and has been cutting back on high-fat foods. Although she has lost some weight overall, she is still unhappy with the shape and size of her breasts.

Suzy's regimen

▶ *Suzy should do exercises that are targeted particularly at the chest muscles. By toning the pectorals supporting the breasts, she can gain a fuller and firmer bust. Exercises that would be especially suitable include the pec dec, incline dumbbell press, and fly.*

▶ *To maintain her general level of fitness but better target her chest muscles, Suzy should take up a sport like tennis or swimming.*

SHAPE CHALLENGE
A sunken chest

Some men develop a flat-chested or sunken physique in which the abdomen protrudes farther than the chest. This condition is usually due to lack of tone in the pectoral muscles. The appearance is made worse by excess body fat around the abdominal area. Young men should remember that they will continue to develop physically until about age 25, so an 18-year-old's expectations of a well-developed chest may be unrealistic. With some attention to exercise and diet, however, major improvements in shape and strength can be achieved relatively easily.

CASE HISTORY

Tony is a 20-year-old college student who is unhappy with his lack of chest development. He eats plenty of food but hardly ever seems to put on weight in the right areas and is finding his abdomen is better defined than his chest. Tony thinks he gets plenty of exercise because he plays basketball for his school. He is aware that he possibly drinks too much but believes he is burning off most of his calories.

Tony's regimen

▶ *Tony would benefit from some specific chest-strengthening exercises. Because he is young and fit, he should be able to do 20 push-ups three times a week. Working out with dumbbells could also help him reach his shape goals faster.*

▶ *Tony's diet could be improved by cutting back on high-fat food and alcohol. This would prevent him from storing excess fat around his stomach.*

Exercises to target the chest

*Tight, restricted chest muscles can contribute to a round-shouldered posture;
to prevent this condition, the pectoral muscles must be stretched regularly. Because
the pectoralis major runs in three different directions, a variety of stretches and exercises
should be done to strengthen the muscle as a whole. Many of the chest exercises also
work other muscles in the upper body, such as the deltoid at the shoulder joint.*

CHEST AND SHOULDER STRETCHES

Stand tall with feet hip width apart. Lock your fingers together behind your back, contract the abdominal muscles, and soften the knees. Gently ease the elbows up and away from the body until you feel the stretch across the chest and shoulders. At the same time, try not to lean forward. Hold the stretch for 20 to 30 seconds, breathing easily.

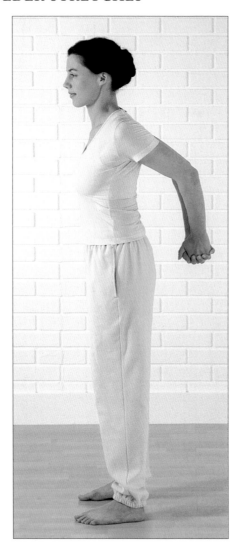

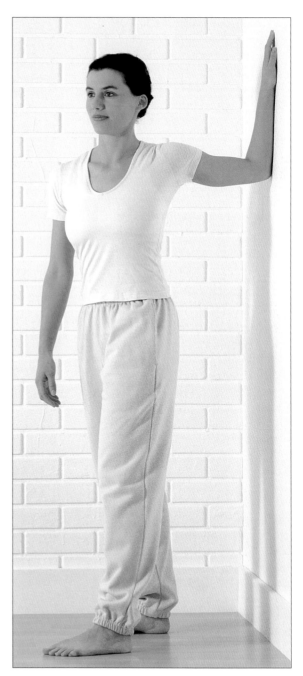

Deep stretch ▶
Place the palm of your hand flat against a wall with the arm at a right angle to your body. Rotate your body away from the arm until you feel a stretch in the chest and front of the shoulder. Hold for 20 to 30 seconds, breathing easily. Change arms.

PUSH-UPS: *Work pectorals, front deltoids, and triceps.*

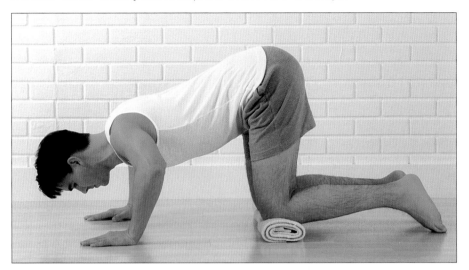

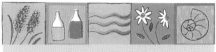

ALMOND OIL

One of the most important of the natural moisturizers is almond oil, extracted from the kernels of sweet, ripe almonds. You can add it to a moisturizer or use it as a massage oil.

To make a gentle exfoliator for the tender skin of the breasts, mix together 1 oz of ground oatmeal with the same amount of finely ground almonds and 1 tbsp of almond oil. Massage the mixture gently onto the breasts and then rinse them thoroughly.

Beginner's easy push-up
Start on your hands and knees. If necessary, rest your knees on a mat or towel for comfort. Your hands should be facing forward under your shoulders.

Keeping abdominal muscles contracted, bend your elbows and lower your chest slowly to the floor, inhaling as you go. Push up to starting position, exhaling. Timing: 4 seconds down, 4 seconds up.

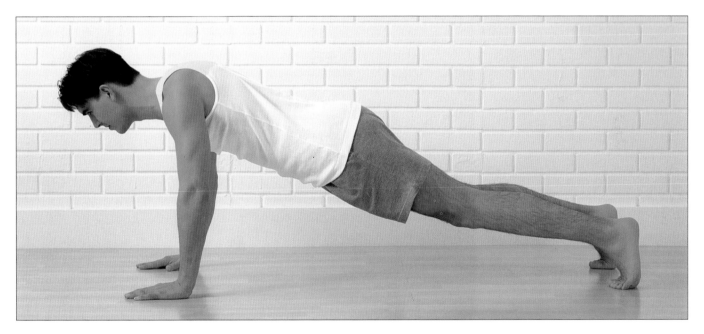

Advanced push-up
To increase the intensity of the beginner's push-up, come up from your knees onto your toes, distributing your weight over your hands and feet. Placing your feet a little wider apart will help you maintain your balance. With abdominal muscles contracted, bend your elbows out to a 90° angle and lower your chest toward the floor, inhaling as you go. Press back up to the starting position, exhaling.

Don't let your abdominal muscles sag because this places stress on the vertebrae of the lower back and can lead to injury. Keep your back straight at all times.

Don't lift your head up too high. This places strain on the neck and can also result in injury.

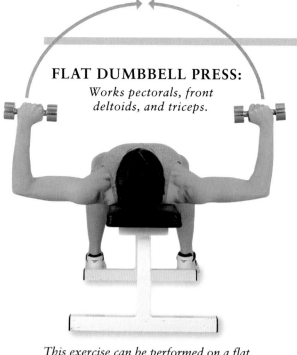

FLAT DUMBBELL PRESS:

Works pectorals, front deltoids, and triceps.

This exercise can be performed on a flat or inclined bench. Inclining the bench will make the exercise slightly easier. Keep the abdominal muscles contracted and lower your back flat onto a bench or step. Assume the starting position, as shown above, with arms bent at 90° to your body. Lift the dumbbells in an arc above your chest until they almost touch. Return to the starting position.

INCLINE DUMBBELL PRESS

Assume the starting position as for the flat dumbbell press but on an incline bench. Lift the dumbbells in an arc above your chest until they almost touch, exhaling as you do so. Lower the weights through the same range, inhaling. Lower only to a position of mild stretch.

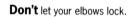

Don't let your elbows lock.

Don't let the dumbbells fall back over the head. This causes the back to arch and may result in injury.

Don't lift the dumbbells too quickly. Use a timing of 4 seconds up, 4 seconds down. Keep the dumbbells evenly weighted in each hand.

INCLINE BENCH FLY

As with the flat dumbbell press, this exercise can be performed on a flat or inclined bench. If you are inclining the bench, assume the starting position as for the flat bench fly. Lift the dumbbells in an arc above your chest until your knuckles almost touch, exhaling as you do so. Lower the weights through the same range, inhaling. Lower only to a position of mild stretch.

FLAT BENCH FLY:

Works pectorals and front deltoids.

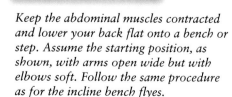

Keep the abdominal muscles contracted and lower your back flat onto a bench or step. Assume the starting position, as shown, with arms open wide but with elbows soft. Follow the same procedure as for the incline bench flyes.

PEC DEC: *Works pectorals and front deltoids.*

You can adjust this machine to increase or reduce the weight you are working with, so check the weight stack before you begin and adjust for your preferred intensity. You can also adjust the height of the seat so that your shoulders and arms are working at the correct angle—approximately 90°. As a beginner you should perform one set of 10 to 20 repetitions for the first four weeks, building up to three sets by week 9.

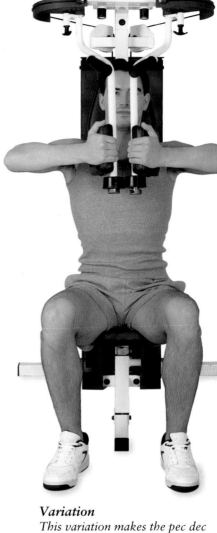

1 *Start with a light, overhand grip. Keep your back straight against the support, your chest lifted, your abdominal muscles contracted, and your feet flat on the floor. Place your forearms flat against the pads with your hands relaxed. Breathe in.*

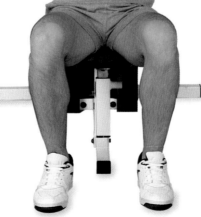

2 *Exhaling, squeeze the pads together in a controlled movement that ends in front of your face. Inhaling, slowly return the pads to the starting position. Timing: 4 seconds in, 4 seconds back.*

Variation
This variation makes the pec dec easier for people with shoulder problems. Grip the two elbow pads as shown; perform the exercise as for steps 1 and 2 at left, making sure your elbows do not lock.

The Back

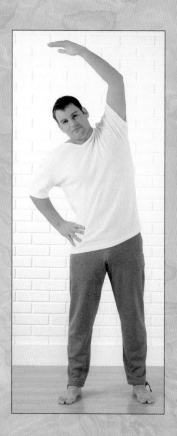

A strong back is vital for almost every activity we perform, from lifting to carrying to walking, and yet back pain is one of the most common complaints. Regular back-strengthening exercises can do much to prevent back problems.

Every movement of your body is dependent on the health of the muscles in your back; even the slightest injury or weakness can lead to incapacitating pain. (At least 80 percent of Americans have suffered back pain at some point in their lives, and for 15 percent the pain is chronic.) It makes sense to include regular stretching and toning of the muscles of the back as an integral feature of an exercise program.

The anatomy of the back
The trapezius—upper, middle, and lower—is the largest of the back muscles. It is roughly diamond

shaped and extends from the base of the skull to the lowest thoracic vertebrae and across the full width of the back and shoulder, where it is attached to both shoulder blades and collarbones. The way in which the trapezius is attached enables it to perform many different actions. The upper trapezius helps support the head and neck, shrugs the shoulders, and stabilizes the shoulders for carrying heavy loads. The middle and lower trapezius stabilize the shoulder blades and retract, or brace, the shoulders during arm movements.

The rhomboid muscles, connected to the upper vertebrae and the

COMPLEMENTARY EXERCISES FOR THE BACK

▶ Swimming is an excellent activity for developing strong back muscles.

▶ Rowing not only counts as one of the best general forms of exercise you can perform but also specifically strengthens the back.

▶ Most forms of gardening, including digging, using a fork, and moving a wheelbarrow, strengthen the back, although good posture is also vital.

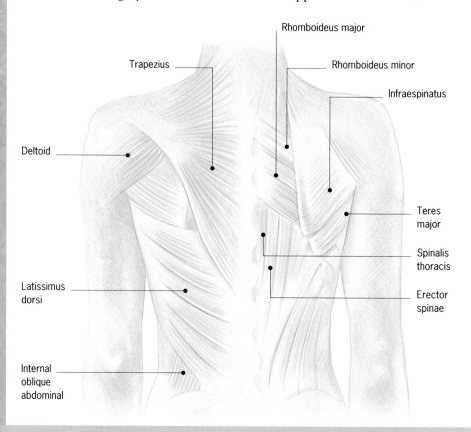

Rhomboideus major

Trapezius

Rhomboideus minor

Infraespinatus

Deltoid

Teres major

Spinalis thoracis

Latissimus dorsi

Erector spinae

Internal oblique abdominal

shoulder blades, work with the middle and lower trapezius. Their job is to brace the shoulder blades.

The two latissimus dorsi are powerful triangular muscles found on either side of the lower back. One side of each muscle is connected to the pelvis and the lower thoracic vertebrae, while the other is attached to the back of the upper arm. Each of these muscles moves an upper arm through a wide range of movements. The main action involves pulling the raised arm down to the side of the body (adduction) against resistance. Acting in reverse, with the arm fixed, the muscle pulls the trunk toward the arm, as when pulling up on a chinning bar.

Back problems

Two common back problems are upper and lower crossed syndromes, which put stress on the vertebrae and intervertebral discs. In the case of upper crossed syndrome, the pectoral and upper trapezius muscles are tight, while the rhomboids and deep neck flexors are weak. With lower crossed syndrome the hip flexors and lower back extensors tighten, while the abdominal muscles and buttocks (gluteals) weaken. With both syndromes bad posture and pain often result. This muscular stress also alters the muscles' normal mechanics and can cause irreversible damage. Where the vertebrae rub together, degeneration may occur, leading to osteoarthritis.

Altered vertebral alignment in the lower back can also place uneven stress on the intervertebral discs. With repeated wear and tear, the discs may rupture (prolapse), placing pressure on the nerve roots and leading to sciatica, in which a sharp pain is felt in the leg.

Regularly exercising and paying proper attention to posture and alignment are vital for the health of your back. The Alexander technique (see pages 47–48) can help with long-standing posture problems.

SHAPE CHALLENGE
Lower crossed syndrome

People with a poor sitting posture can develop the condition called lower crossed syndrome, which is one of the most common causes of lower back pain. As the lumbar spine is pulled forward, the intervertebral discs are compressed and the vertebrae rub together, causing pain.

Because so many occupations are now primarily sedentary, this problem is becoming increasingly widespread, but exercise can bring about major improvements.

CASE HISTORY
Mary is a 48-year-old receptionist in a government housing agency. Most of her day is spent at her desk, answering the phone, greeting visitors, and typing. Over the past few months she has developed lower back pain. Her doctor has recommended that she take regular breaks to stretch her back throughout the working day, but because her desk must always be manned, Mary finds it virtually impossible to do so.

Mary's regimen
▶ *It is essential that Mary start stretching her hip flexors and lower back extensors every morning and evening to restore them to a normal length. She can then strengthen her abdominal muscles with crunches and her gluteals with lunges. She should also develop endurance in the lower back extensors using exercises such as superman.*

▶ *Mary should improve her seated posture, perhaps with an Alexander technique therapist. Sitting with her spine straight and shoulders back will be beneficial.*

SHAPE CHALLENGE
Upper crossed syndrome

Incorrect training, in which the chest muscles are overworked while little attention is paid to the upper back, can lead to a common pattern of muscular imbalances called upper crossed syndrome. This condition is often seen simply as a case of poor posture—chin projected forward and shoulders rounded. It may lead to shoulder and neck pain or injury during many normal movements, and so the problem should be addressed.

CASE HISTORY
Michael is a 45-year-old self-employed plumber. Having become concerned recently about his expanding waistline and sagging pectorals, Michael joined a gym. He has concentrated on working his chest muscles in order to improve his chest shape. Although he's been attending the gym for two months now and has also made changes in his diet, he's been disappointed to see that his stomach still looks larger than his chest.

Michael's regimen
▶ *Michael needs to redirect his training toward the muscles of the upper back to balance his physique. He should begin by regularly stretching the upper trapezius and pectorals until they reach a desirable length. To help return the shoulders to a neutral position, he should train his weakened rhomboids with exercises such as the seated row, single arm dumbbell row, or reverse fly.*

▶ *He should also examine his posture for signs of weakness that could be affecting his shape.*

Exercises to target the back

Stretching the back is absolutely vital before beginning any form of exercise. If you fail to stretch properly, you could easily strain a muscle, causing pain and even immobility. It is also important to have a comfortable exercise mat to work on to avoid pressing on sensitive spinal nerves. Mats are readily available in most sporting goods stores.

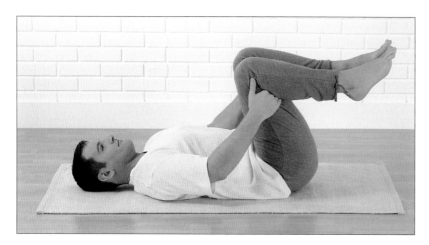

BACK STRETCHES

Lower back stretch

Lying on your back, grip your legs underneath your knees at the back of your thighs and ease the legs in toward the body. Keep your body aligned and your head and neck relaxed. Hold the stretch for 10 to 20 seconds, breathing easily all the time. For a variation on this stretch, rest your lower legs on a chair with hips and knees at a 90° angle to the body.

Lower back rotation stretch

1 *Lie on your back with your whole body aligned. Stretch out your arms at shoulder height. Bend one leg, keeping the foot flat on the floor.*

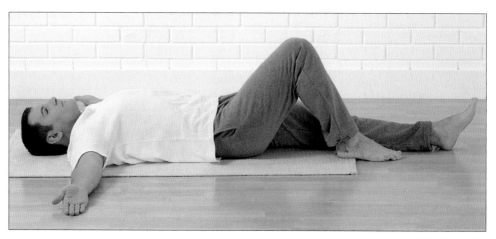

2 *Bring the bent knee across the midline of the body, allowing it to fall slowly to the opposite side; stop when you feel a comfortable stretch. If desired, place your hand on your outer thigh and apply gentle pressure to increase the stretch. Hold the stretch 10 to 20 seconds, then relax, return to the starting position, and repeat on the other side. For a variation you can perform this stretch by bending both knees together. Then slowly ease both knees down to the floor, first to the left and then to the right.*

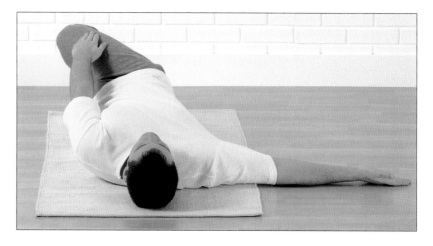

SEATED ROW: *Works rhomboids and latissimus dorsi.*

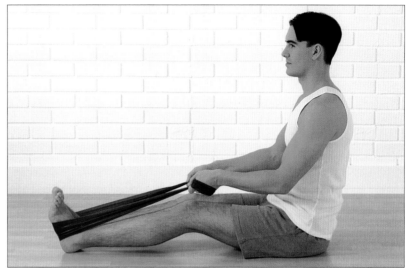

1 *An elastic band is needed for this exercise. Sit on the floor with legs extended in front of you and knees slightly bent. Make sure that your* back is straight and abdominal muscles are contracted. Pull the elastic band with your arms until there is a slight tension in the band.

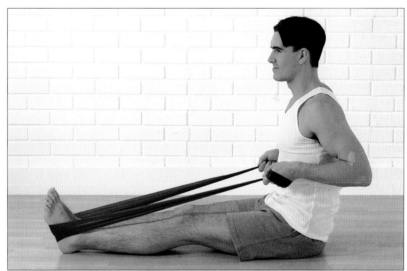

2 *Squeeze your elbows slowly backward, increasing the tension in the elastic band. Exhale as you do this. Inhale as you return slowly to* the starting position. Keep your back straight and abdominal muscles contracted throughout the movement.

Don't lean back too far and allow your back to arch because this will place stress on your lower back.

Don't lift your shoulders up toward your ears; this may cause pain in the neck.

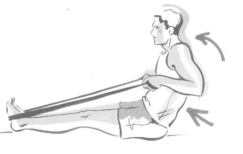

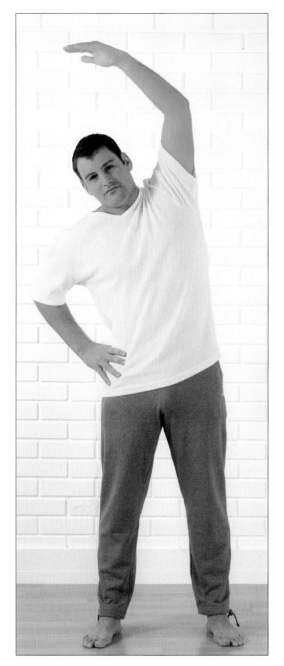

Latissimus dorsi stretch

Stand with feet hip width apart, your abdominal muscles contracted, and one arm straight overhead. Lean sideways from the hip joint but keep the hips level. Extend your raised arm until you feel a stretch. Hold the stretch for 10 to 20 seconds, breathing easily throughout. Repeat the stretch on the other side.

SINGLE ARM DUMBBELL ROW: *Works rhomboids and latissimus dorsi.*

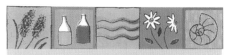

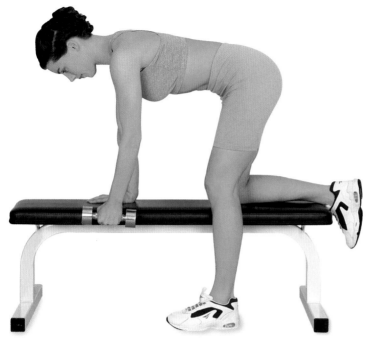

TEA TREE OIL

Tea tree oil has become more appreciated as a medicinal oil in recent years. Extracted from the leaves and twigs of an Australian tree, it is a powerful antiseptic and natural antibiotic that can be very useful for a range of skin problems, including acne.

The back can be susceptible to acne, particularly in people who exercise regularly, because it is difficult to properly clean and exfoliate the area. Making up a back scrub containing tea tree oil and using a long-handled brush to apply it can help keep acne under control. You can also ask your partner or a friend to apply the scrub for you.

1 *For this exercise you will need a bench or step and a dumbbell. Support your body weight equally with one leg and arm on the bench, as shown.*

It is important to keep a slight bend in the leg that is standing. Keep your abdominal muscles contracted and your back horizontal.

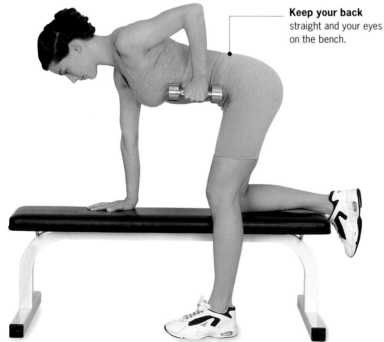

Keep your back straight and your eyes on the bench.

Don't lift up your head. This action places stress on the back of the neck and may cause injury.

Don't let the abdominal muscles sag. This places strain on the lower back.

Don't let the knee of the leg that is standing lock.

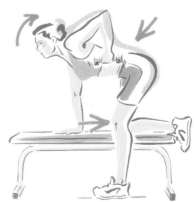

2 *Lift the dumbbell upward, keeping your elbow close to your side, and breathe out. Slowly return to the starting position while inhaling. Your speed of*

movement should be 4 seconds up and 4 seconds down. Repeat the exercise up to 10 times before switching sides to exercise the other arm.

SUPERMAN: *Works upper and lower back extensors and gluteals.*

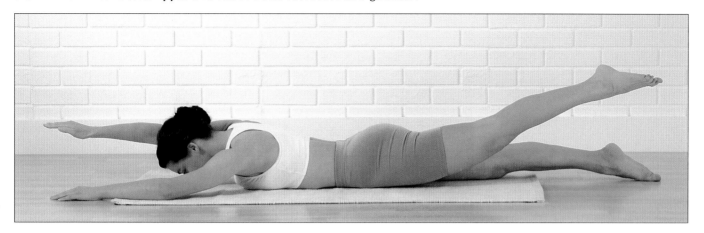

Lie on your abdomen with your whole body in line and a slight bend in your elbows and knees. Keep your head and neck relaxed. Lift opposite arm and leg together in a slow, controlled movement, raising your leg to a comfortable height. Hold briefly and squeeze the buttocks. Breathe out. Lower your leg slowly and with control, inhaling as you finish. Repeat with the other arm and leg.

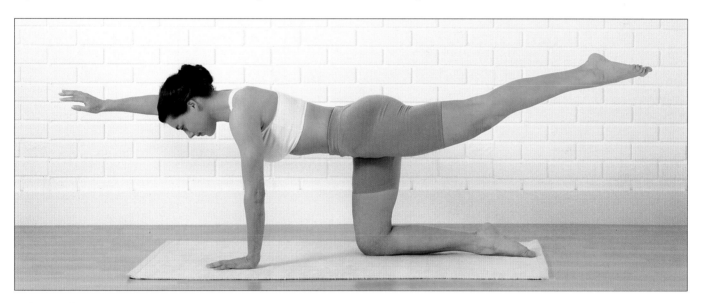

Advanced position
To increase the intensity of the superman exercise, come up onto all fours with knees hip width apart and hands at shoulder width. Keeping elbows unlocked, spine straight, and eyes facing down, slowly raise the right arm and left leg until horizontal; do not allow knees and elbows to lock. Squeeze buttocks briefly at the top. Repeat with the other arm and leg.

Don't allow your hip to rise from the mat because this places the lower back in a strained, twisted position.

Don't allow your neck to crane backward because this strains the spine and neck.

Don't allow your knee to bend excessively. Move smoothly to the up position—don't jerk.

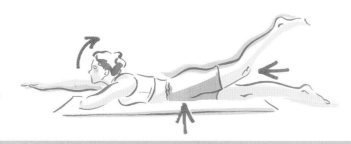

LATERAL PULL-DOWN: *Works the latissimus dorsi.*

Before beginning this exercise, check the weight load in the pin stack and adjust the seat level to your height. This machine also develops strength in the arms, specifically the biceps.

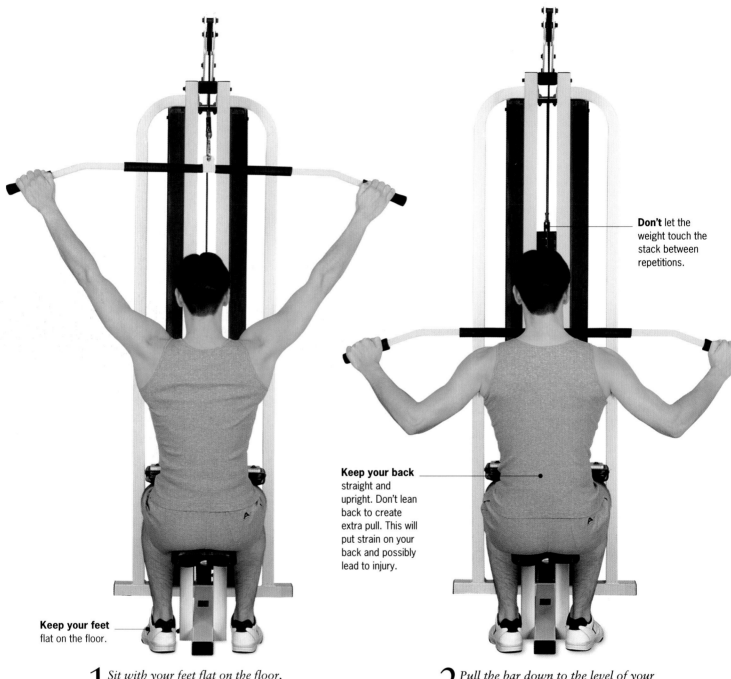

Don't let the weight touch the stack between repetitions.

Keep your back straight and upright. Don't lean back to create extra pull. This will put strain on your back and possibly lead to injury.

Keep your feet flat on the floor.

1 *Sit with your feet flat on the floor, abdominal muscles contracted, and your back straight. Your lower body is stabilized by the leg pad, which rests on your thighs. Use a wide overhand grip.*

2 *Pull the bar down to the level of your upper chest, exhaling. Squeeze your back muscles at the bottom position. Slowly return the bar to the starting position, inhaling. Timing: 4 seconds down, 4 seconds up. Start with one set of 10 to 20 repetitions of the exercise in the first four weeks, building up to three sets by week 9.*

REVERSE FLY:

Works rhomboids, deltoids, latissimus dorsi, and biceps.

1 *Sit with your feet together, keeping the abdominal muscles contracted and the back flat. Lean forward. Begin with the dumbbells underneath your legs and your elbows slightly bent.*

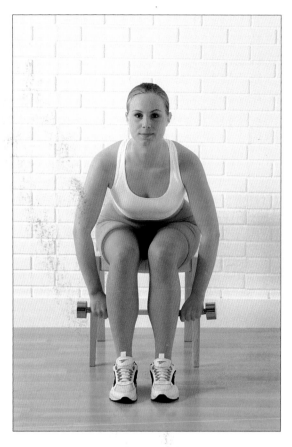

2 *Squeeze your elbows upward and backward until they are parallel to your body at shoulder height. Hold briefly at the top and then return to the starting position in a slow, controlled movement. Keep your neck relaxed throughout the exercise.*

Variation

If you have shoulder problems, you will find this variation on the pull-down easier. Grip the bar with your palms facing backward and pull it down until it is level with the upper chest. Squeeze back muscles at the bottom position. Return the bar to the starting position in a controlled movement.

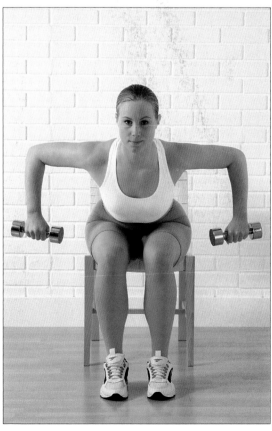

Arms and Hands

Strength in the arms and hands is essential for a wide range of daily activities, from performing chores to enjoying your favorite leisure pursuits. It is relatively easy to target the relevant muscles to achieve improvements rapidly.

Both men and women can quickly lose muscle tone and strength in the arms, particularly the biceps. Not using these muscles for any extended period of time will cause them to waste to some degree, which will affect both your appearance and the ease with which you do daily chores.

The anatomy of the arm

The main muscles of the upper arms are the deltoid, biceps, and triceps. Although these muscles have their own individual functions, they are often used to assist the larger chest and back muscles during a number of activities.

The deltoid is a V-shaped muscle that originates at the collarbone and the top of the shoulder blade and is connected to the side of the upper arm. It is divided into three parts—front, middle, and rear—each of which performs distinct actions.

The middle deltoid, the most powerful of the three, is mainly responsible for raising the arm from the side of the body (abduction). The front deltoid assists the upper pectoral in lifting the arm in front of the body. Working in conjunction with the rhomboids, the rear deltoid pulls the arm backward from in front of the body.

COMPLEMENTARY EXERCISES FOR THE ARMS AND HANDS

▶ Rock climbing is a good sport for developing arm and hand strength. You don't have to climb outdoors; indoor climbing centers, which are increasingly popular, are an excellent and safe way to develop your expertise.

▶ Martial arts place great emphasis on arm strength and flexibility. Judo, karate, and aikido, as well as gentler forms such as t'ai chi, will all help you build strength.

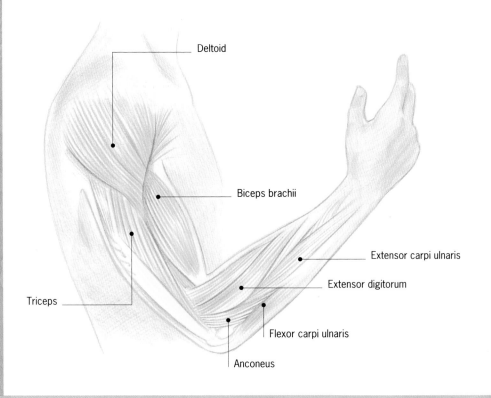

Deltoid

Biceps brachii

Extensor carpi ulnaris

Extensor digitorum

Triceps

Flexor carpi ulnaris

Anconeus

The biceps (biceps brachii) covers the front of the upper arm. Its main functions are to bring the forearm toward the shoulder, as when eating, and to turn the hand palm up, as when turning a doorknob—a movement called supination. The muscle contracts powerfully when carrying heavy weights.

The triceps covers the whole back of the upper arm. Its main function is to straighten the elbow joint from a bent position (extension), but only when the movement takes place against resistance or gravity, for instance, when pushing something away from yourself. When you slowly lower the forearm, the triceps muscle is relaxing while the biceps is contracting.

Anatomy of the hand

The muscles of the hand and fingers require precise control to carry out their numerous functions. These muscles can be broadly divided into those that bend and extend the wrist (flexors and extensors) and those that cause the hand to rotate palm up or palm down (supinators and pronators). Within the hand many small muscles produce the combined movements of the fingers and thumb, as when making a fist.

Arm and hand problems

A number of common muscular problems result from using muscles incorrectly. Tennis elbow, characterized by pain and tenderness on the outside of the elbow and in the back of the forearm, is an inflammation of the tendon that attaches the extensor muscles to the humerus, the bone of the upper arm. Playing racquet sports with a poor grip or doing such activities as gardening can bring on the condition. Rest is often advised as part of treatment, but addressing muscle usage is also important. Perhaps the most common problem experienced in the arm, wrist, or hand is repetitive strain injury.

SHAPE CHALLENGE
Flabby arms

In women a major site of fat storage, especially in later life, is the back of the arms around the triceps. The amount of fat stored there depends on overall body fat and on genetic and hormonal factors. If body fat levels are high, toning exercises alone will have little influence on arm shape (remember that muscles lie underneath the visible body fat). Body fat must be reduced with a program of diet and aerobic exercise, and toning work will then show some results.

CASE HISTORY

Dorothy is 55 years old and has recently retired from work as a nurse's aide. Her job was quite demanding physically, involving some heavy lifting and cleaning duties, but now that she has retired, Dorothy feels entitled to a break and has been fairly inactive. After a few weeks of relaxation, Dorothy decided to rejoin her local bowling club and was shocked to discover how weak her upper arms were and how quickly she tired; she was also very sore after each session.

Dorothy's regimen

▶ *Dorothy has already lost much of the upper arm strength she developed while working. She must recognize that she will need some form of exercise to maintain muscle strength during her retirement. Bowling will be helpful in the long run, but initially she will need to rebuild strength by performing specific exercises, such as the dumbbell lateral raise and the triceps dip. She may also have to reassess her diet and cut back on excess fat intake.*

SHAPE CHALLENGE
Repetitive strain

Although mainly associated with keyboard operators and assembly line workers, repetitive strain injury can affect anyone who repeatedly uses particular muscles in their occupation. Musicians are commonly affected, the thumb and fingers being a source of problems, particularly for players of woodwind instruments. Symptoms include pain and stiffness in the affected joint. Although rest is necessary to ease the problem, this is impractical for long periods.

CASE HISTORY

Robert is 40 years old and a member of a jazz group in which he plays the flute. The group members are thrilled that their bookings have recently increased, and from being part-time hobbyists, they now appear on the verge of becoming commercially successful. Robert has given up his part-time job in a local library to concentrate on his music but is distressed to find that his playing has become severely hampered by stiffness and pain in his fingers.

Robert's regimen

▶ *Robert's hands did not have sufficient time to adjust to the new demands placed on them. He needs to introduce a program of regular stretching to warm and loosen his muscles before he begins practicing each day. Squeezing a tennis ball every day can help him develop strength in the other muscles of the fingers.*

▶ *Robert should also take some breaks from his music. An activity like t'ai chi would be relaxing and might help ease his muscle strain.*

Exercises to target the arms

Even if you exercise your arm muscles regularly through daily activities, specific exercises can help you improve areas of weakness. After just a few weeks of strengthening work, you should notice improvement in your ability to carry out everyday activities, such as toting shopping bags, doing household chores, and getting out of a chair.

ARM STRETCHES

Triceps stretch

This stretch can be done in a sitting or standing position. With abdominal muscles contracted and back straight, place the fingers of one hand between your shoulder blades. Support this arm with the other hand as shown. With the supporting arm placed near the back of the head, apply pressure to the elbow, pushing it down your spine and breathing evenly all the time. You should feel a stretch in the back of the arm. Repeat for the other side.

If this stretch is very uncomfortable, do it with the supporting arm near the front of the head and push the arm from lower down on the elbow.

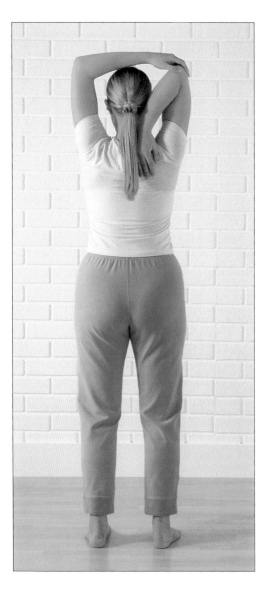

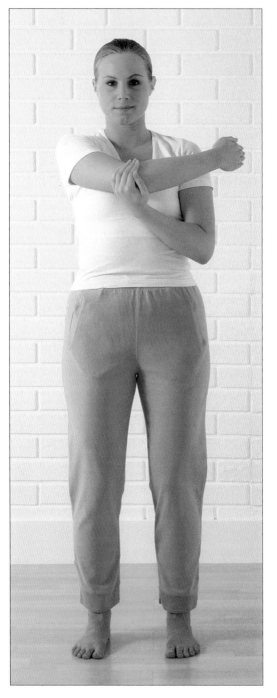

Shoulder stretch ▶

Stand with feet hip width apart, abdominal muscles contracted, and knees slightly bent. Bring one arm across your front at shoulder height. Support the arm at the elbow with the other hand and ease the arm farther across the body until you feel a stretch in the shoulder.

BICEPS CURL

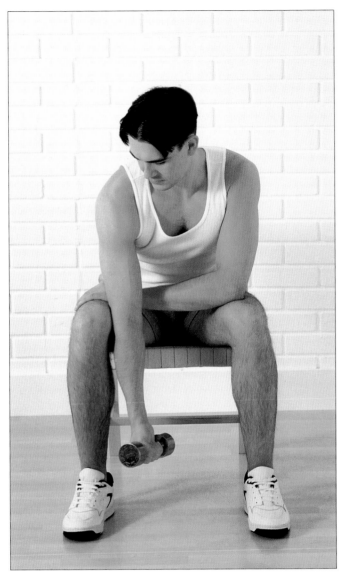

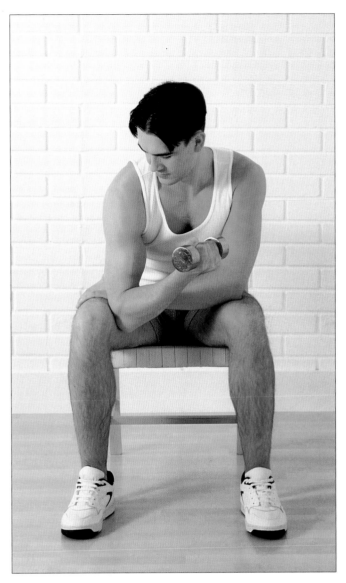

1 Sit on a bench or chair with feet slightly wider than hip width apart. With your abdominal muscles contracted, lean slightly forward with your back straight. Slowly straighten the arm carrying the dumbbell toward the floor, keeping it supported at the elbow by the other arm and the inner thigh.

2 Moving only the exercising arm, squeeze the dumbbell upward until level with your shoulder, exhaling as you go. Briefly squeeze your biceps at the top position. In a slow, controlled movement, lower your arm to the starting position.

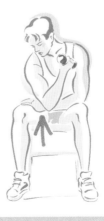

Don't allow your elbow to lose contact with your inner thigh and supporting arm. This makes the exercise much less effective.

DUMBBELL LATERAL RAISE: *Works the deltoids.*

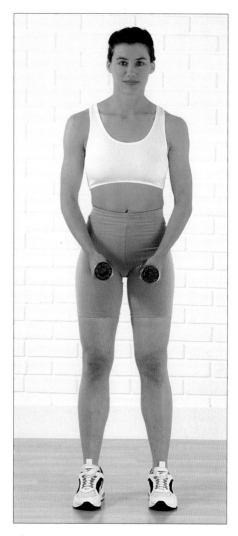

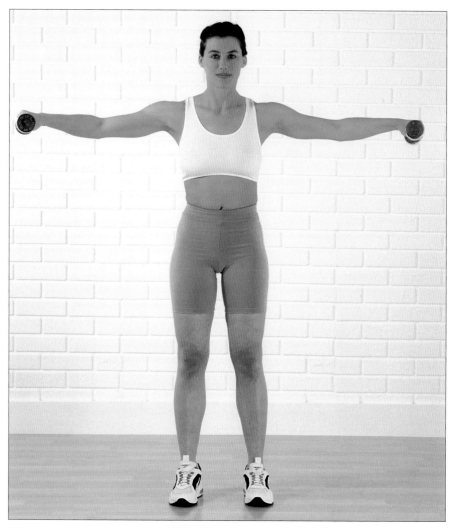

1 *Stand with abdominal muscles contracted, back straight, and knees slightly bent. Start with the dumbbells lowered together in front of your body and a small bend in the elbows.*

2 *Lift the dumbbells sideways away from your body until your arms are level with your shoulders, exhaling as you do so. In a slow and controlled*

movement, lower the weights to the starting position, inhaling. If possible, do this exercise in front of a mirror to check your technique and body symmetry.

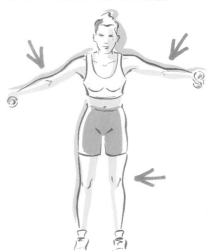

Don't lean forward with knees locked because this can put excessive strain on the lower back. Arms should be level; use a mirror to check correct arm height and symmetry.

Don't allow elbows to lock; this can strain the elbow joint.

SHOULDER PRESS: *Works the deltoids and triceps.*

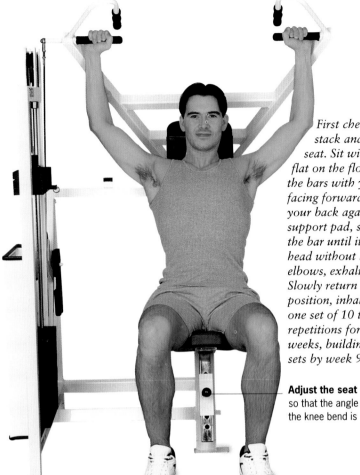

First check the weight stack and adjust the seat. Sit with your feet flat on the floor and grip the bars with your palms facing forward. Keeping your back against the support pad, slowly raise the bar until it is over your head without locking your elbows, exhaling as you go. Slowly return to the starting position, inhaling. Start with one set of 10 to 20 repetitions for the first 4 weeks, building to three sets by week 9.

Adjust the seat
so that the angle of
the knee bend is 90°.

SANDALWOOD

Sandalwood essential oil is good for soothing irritated and inflamed skin conditions. It has been valued as a cosmetic from early times and was a very important spice in the trade of the Dutch East India Company.

Regular exercise can lead to rough, hard, or irritated skin, which sandalwood-based lotions and creams can help to heal. Recent evidence suggests that sandalwood helps to increase the turnover of surface skin cells, leading to a fresher complexion.

MACHINE TRICEPS DIP

Grasp the handles with an overhand grip. Exhaling, push the handles in a slow, controlled movement until they are level with the seat of the machine. Inhaling, slowly return to the starting position. Start with one set of 10 to 20 repetitions for the first 4 weeks, building to three sets by week 9.

If there are rollers, place your
legs in front of the first and
behind the second; they serve
to keep your legs still.

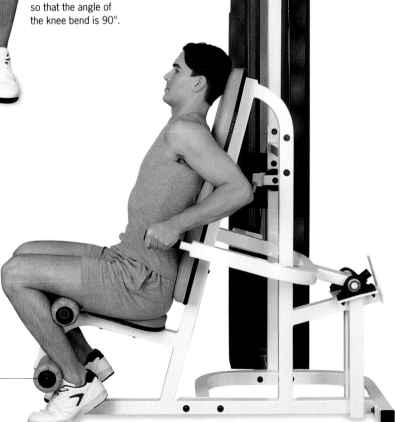

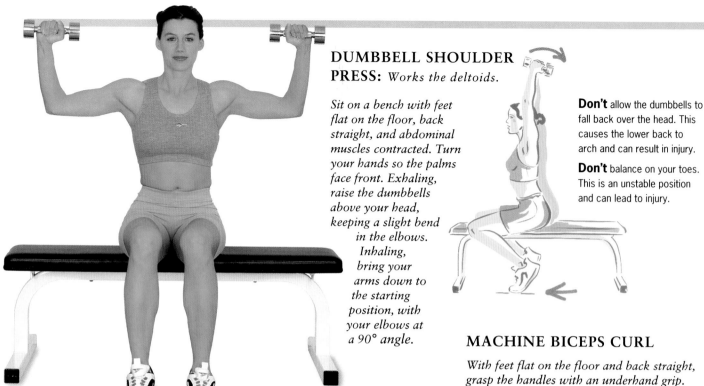

DUMBBELL SHOULDER PRESS: *Works the deltoids.*

Sit on a bench with feet flat on the floor, back straight, and abdominal muscles contracted. Turn your hands so the palms face front. Exhaling, raise the dumbbells above your head, keeping a slight bend in the elbows. Inhaling, bring your arms down to the starting position, with your elbows at a 90° angle.

Don't allow the dumbbells to fall back over the head. This causes the lower back to arch and can result in injury.

Don't balance on your toes. This is an unstable position and can lead to injury.

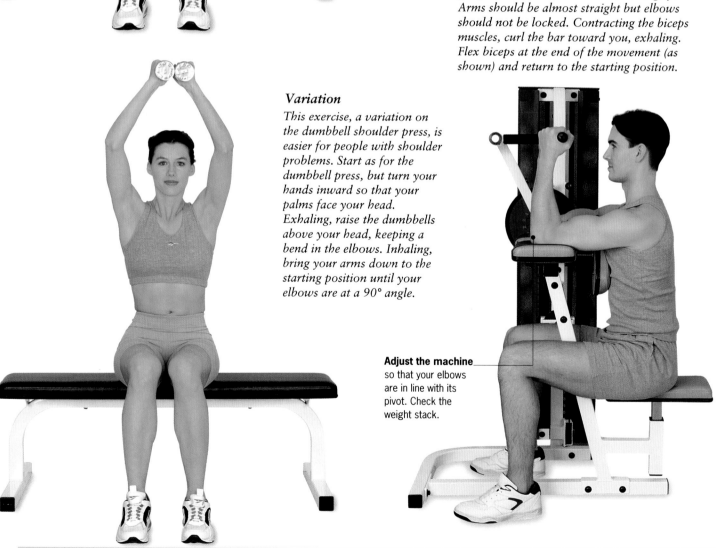

Variation

This exercise, a variation on the dumbbell shoulder press, is easier for people with shoulder problems. Start as for the dumbbell press, but turn your hands inward so that your palms face your head. Exhaling, raise the dumbbells above your head, keeping a bend in the elbows. Inhaling, bring your arms down to the starting position until your elbows are at a 90° angle.

MACHINE BICEPS CURL

With feet flat on the floor and back straight, grasp the handles with an underhand grip. Arms should be almost straight but elbows should not be locked. Contracting the biceps muscles, curl the bar toward you, exhaling. Flex biceps at the end of the movement (as shown) and return to the starting position.

Adjust the machine so that your elbows are in line with its pivot. Check the weight stack.

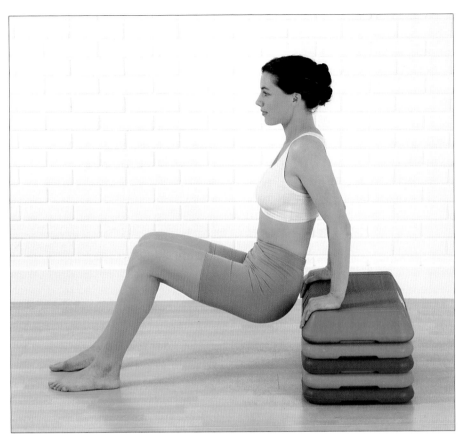

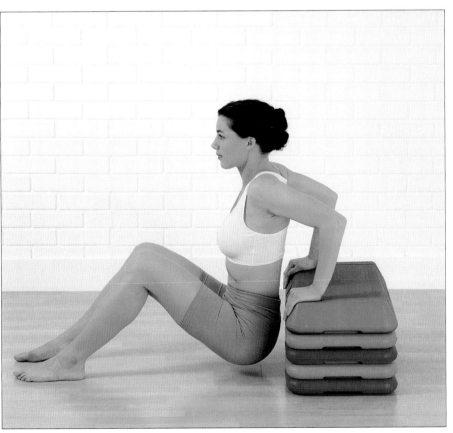

TRICEPS DIP

1 *Place your hands facing forward on a step or bench, shoulder width apart, so that your arms support your body weight. Place your feet shoulder width apart, keeping a bend in your knees and feet flat on the floor. It is important that the step or bench be at the correct height. If the step is too low, the exercise will not be effective because you will not be fully extending the triceps muscles. If, on the other hand, the step is too high, your body will be at too extreme an angle.*

2 *Inhaling, slowly lower your body by bending the elbows but not beyond a 90° angle. If you experience shoulder pain, bend only to a comfortable position. Keep your buttocks close to the step or bench at all times. Push upward to the starting position and exhale. Your elbows should remain slightly bent at the top position.*

Don't place your feet too far away from the step. This will cause the body to lower at an angle and place undue strain on the shoulder joints.

Don't lock the elbows on the up phase of the exercise; maintain a slight bend. On the down phase the arms should be lowered to a 90° angle at the elbow joint.

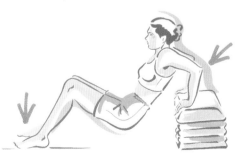

Exercises to target the wrists

You may imagine that your wrists get sufficient exercise from daily activities and that specific strengthening exercises are unnecessary. However, when you consider how important they are to every aspect of life and that the incidence of such problems as repetitive strain injury is on the rise, it makes good sense to give your wrists a daily workout. Most of these exercises can be performed easily at a desk or even while watching television.

WRIST EXERCISES: *Work the extensors and flexors.*

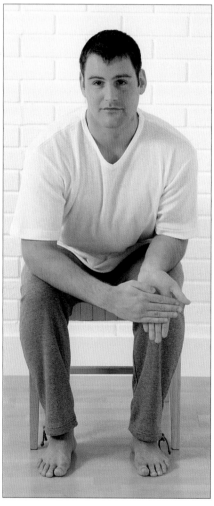 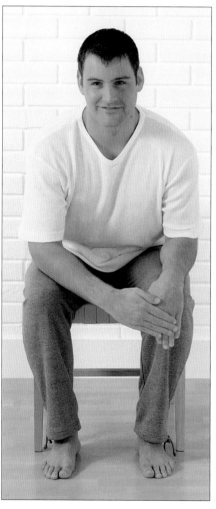 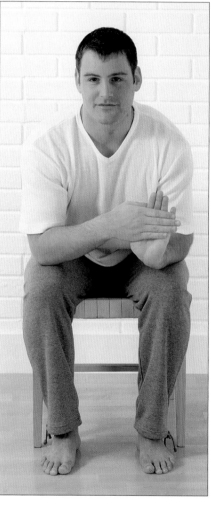

1 *Sit on a chair with your left hand hanging over the edge of your left knee, palm upward. Keep the lower arm in contact with your thigh at all times. Follow the sequence, holding each stretch for 10 to 30 seconds. Start with a flexor stretch: using your right hand to control the movement of the left, bend your hand down until you can feel an easy stretch in the wrist and hand.*

2 *Moving to an extensor stretch, turn your palm so that it faces downward. Apply downward pressure until you can feel an easy stretch in the back of the forearm.*

3 *From this down position, gently ease the hand backward until you can feel the stretch in the inner wrist and back of the hand. Repeat the sequence with the other hand.*

WRIST MOBILITY EXERCISES

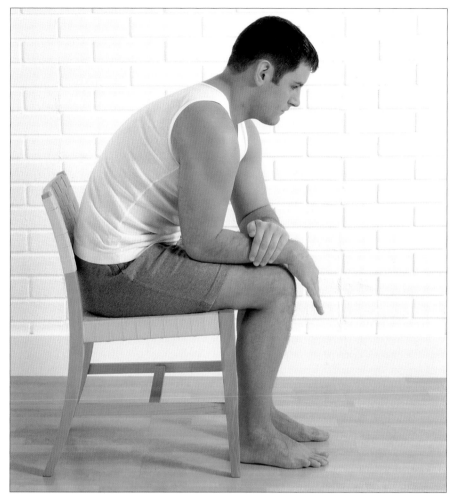

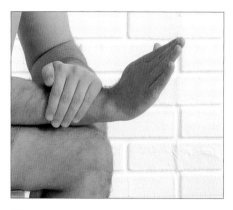

2 *From the down position, ease the hand up as far as it will go so that you feel a gentle stretch. Then turn the hand so that the thumb points upward.*

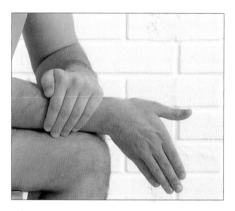

3 *Now bend the hand down sideways, keeping the wrist joint supported on the thigh with the other hand.*

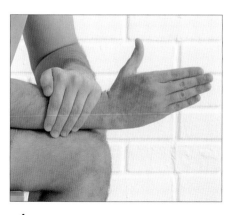

4 *Ease the hand up again as far as it will go until you feel an easy stretch. Slowly return to the starting position.*

1 *Sit on a chair with your right hand hanging over the edge of your right knee, palm facing downward and supported at the wrist by your left hand. Follow the sequence slowly, holding each position for 2 seconds. Repeat the cycle 4 times, then change to the other hand. To increase the intensity, hold a light weight in the hand.*

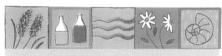

LAVENDER OIL

Lavender oil is an essential oil that helps heal scar tissue and thus is ideal for cuts and burns. Its properties were discovered accidentally by the developer of aromatherapy, René Gattefosse, who found that lavender oil healed a bad burn quickly and without scarring.

Lavender oil is suitable for most skin types except very dry, sensitive skin. To make a healing cuticle cream, add 5 drops of lavender oil and 10 drops of tea tree oil to a base cream.

The Abdomen

In most people the abdominal muscles are relatively weak and overstretched. They usually require strengthening rather than stretching. Toning this area helps improve not only your shape but also your posture and may even relieve back pain.

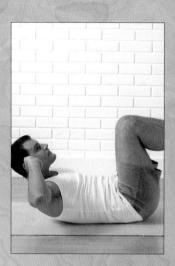

COMPLEMENTARY EXERCISES FOR THE ABDOMEN

► It is essential to build good abdominal tone before doing vigorous activities; if your trunk is unstable, you could injure yourself. Once basic tone is established, however, exercises such as tennis, golf, yoga, and t'ai chi are excellent for maintaining or improving abdominal tone.

► When performed with correct technique, lifting, carrying, gardening, and weight training provide a good abdominal workout.

The abdomen is a common problem area of the body. As a major site of fat storage for both men and women, it is the section where you will probably first notice any weight gain, yet it is often difficult to isolate and target the abdominal muscles when exercising. For example, such exercises as full sit-ups use the abdominal muscles only for the first 30 degrees of the movement; after that, the hip flexors complete the motion. Sit-up exercises can also lead to injury because the hip flexors pull on the spine, altering posture and increasing disc pressure. Any movements that extend the muscles from a prone position are generally unsuitable for people who have back conditions, such as a prolapsed disc, or who have a history of lower back pain. They should consult a doctor or physiotherapist before attempting abdominal exercises.

Pregnancy places particular demands on the muscles of the abdomen, and getting the muscles back to their former strength can be a real challenge.

The anatomy of the abdomen

There are four main abdominal muscles—the rectus abdominis, the internal and external obliques, and the transversus abdominis. Together they provide stability

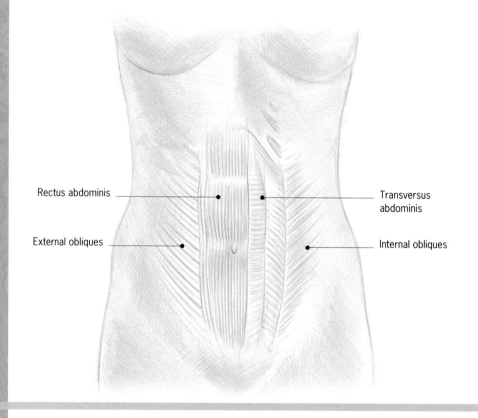

Rectus abdominis

Transversus abdominis

External obliques

Internal obliques

for the trunk and protect and support the digestive organs. The rectus abdominis flexes the trunk by pulling the lower breastbone toward the pelvis—or vice versa. The internal and external obliques work in combination to rotate the trunk. The transversus abdominis compresses the abdominal contents to flatten your abdomen and hold in your stomach. Some abdominal exercises use one or two of these muscles and some use all four.

The abdominal muscles are arranged in layers and are unusual in that they are joined to other muscles by tendons; most skeletal muscles are connected to bone.

Abdominal problems

After pregnancy many women find it difficult to regain the strength of their abdominal muscles. However, if correct abdominal training is done during pregnancy, muscle tone will return more quickly following the birth. This is especially important for women preparing to return to sports or other kinds of exercise. It is also essential to strengthen the muscles of the pelvic floor, which can be weakened after childbirth. The pelvic floor muscles act like a sling to support the pelvic organs; they also help strengthen the sphincter muscle, which controls the flow of urine from the bladder. Weak muscles can lead to urinary incontinence, as well as irritation of the hip and sacroiliac joints.

Another common shape problem is lordotic posture. This results from weak abdominal muscles failing to compress the abdomen adequately, allowing it to protrude forward. The protruding abdomen exerts pull on the lower spine, often leading to back pain or disc problems. Excess body fat in the area worsens the problem. Because the body tends to store more fat in the abdominal area as we grow older, it is particularly important to maintain abdominal tone through exercise.

SHAPE CHALLENGE
A fit pregnancy

During pregnancy the abdominal muscles stretch to allow for the baby to grow. Later on, the hormone relaxin acts on the linea alba—a tendinous sheath that joins the two sides of the rectus abdominis—causing it to soften so that it can stretch sideways, thus providing more room for the baby to grow.

Increasingly, fitness experts are finding that maintaining abdominal tone during her pregnancy can help a woman to regain muscle strength much faster after the birth.

CASE HISTORY

Ruth is a 29-year-old woman who is 20 weeks pregnant with her first child. A keen tennis player, she hopes to be able to return to playing with her club a few months after the birth. So far Ruth's pregnancy has progressed well, with little morning sickness, and she has felt well enough to swim three times a week. However, now that she is starting to grow bigger, she is feeling less confident about her exercise program.

Ruth's regimen

▶ *Ruth first needs to have a thorough checkup with her doctor and discuss her exercise plans. Her doctor will advise her if there are particular exercises to avoid.*

▶ *She should then visit a local gym, where fitness experts can devise an exercise plan to suit her. They may advise her about the safety of doing such abdominal exercises as crunches and oblique curls. They may also recommend aqua aerobics as a gentler alternative to swimming laps.*

SHAPE CHALLENGE
Lordotic posture

General weight gain combined with weak abdominal muscles can lead to the development of lordotic posture, characterized by a potbellied appearance. This condition can also be a common cause of lower back pain. When the abdominal muscles are weak, they allow the abdomen to exert a forward pull on the lower (lumbar) spine. This places stress on the vertebrae and supporting structures, leading to chronic degeneration of the lumbar vertebrae and increased pressure on the vertebral discs.

CASE HISTORY

Barry, who is 57 years old, took early retirement last year. Though he's always been a little overweight, over the past few months he has gained 10 pounds and is embarrassed about his protruding stomach. He enjoys golf, but he has been alarmed to find himself out of breath with only a little exertion on the course and has also suffered painful lower back spasms. His doctor has diagnosed lordotic posture and recommends regular exercise.

Barry's regimen

▶ *Barry must develop an overall health and fitness plan in conjunction with his doctor and a fitness instructor. He must first improve his general level of fitness with some regular aerobic exercise before turning his attention to his abdomen. It will also be essential to change his diet, cutting back on alcohol and high-fat foods.*

▶ *Once Barry's general fitness has improved, he can focus on curls and crunches to strengthen his abdominal muscles.*

Exercises to target the abdomen

The abdominal muscles are the only ones for which stretching is generally not so vital. You should bear in mind , however, that abdominal exercises will also work other muscles of the body, such as the neck, back, legs, and chest, so they should be preceded by a thorough warmup and general stretch routine.

PRONE EXTENSION STRETCH

Lie face down with elbows in line with your shoulders. Keeping hips and feet in contact with the floor and breathing evenly, gently lift your head and chest off the floor and hold for 10 seconds. You will feel a stretch in the abdominal muscles. Repeat 3 times.

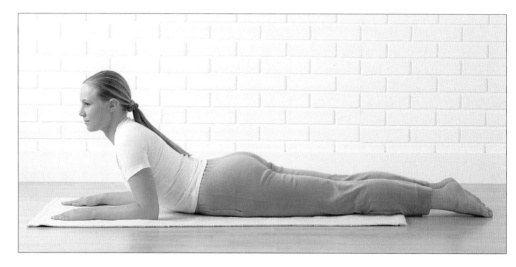

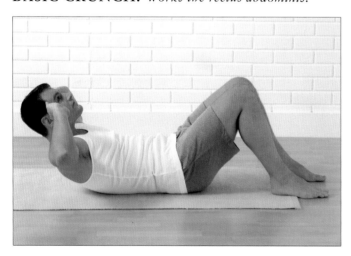

Don't perform this exercise if you have existing back problems.

Don't allow your elbows to lift off the floor. This hyperextended position places strain on the vertebrae of the lower back and may cause damage.

Don't tilt your head backward because this places stress on the vertebrae at the back of the neck and may cause damage.

BASIC CRUNCH: *Works the rectus abdominis.*

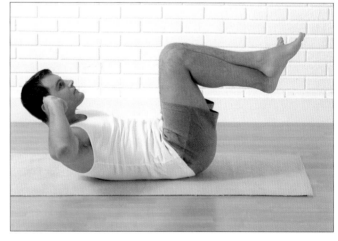

Lie on your back with your knees bent, feet hip width apart, abdominal muscles pulled in, and hands on either side of your head. Exhaling, squeeze up, raising shoulders a little way off the floor. Hold briefly and then slowly ease down, inhaling.

Advanced
Perform this exercise in the same way as the basic crunch, but keep both feet lifted off the floor while raising your shoulders, as shown.

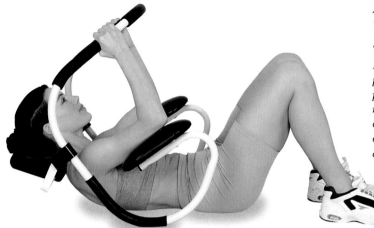

AB TRAINER CRUNCH:
Works rectus abdominis.

This equipment is called an ab trainer. It supports the head and neck while you perform crunches and is very useful for people who experience neck pain during normal crunches. Rest your elbows lightly on the pads and hold the frame with a light overhand grip. Keeping your lower back in contact with the floor, slowly lift your shoulders off the floor, taking the rolling frame with you.

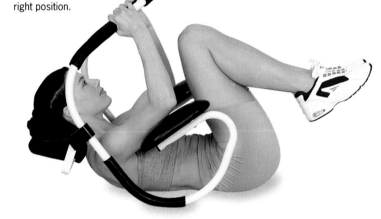

Neck support keeps your head in the right position.

Advanced
Do the basic ab trainer crunch above but lift your legs off the floor at the same time you lift your shoulders. This makes the abdominal muscles work harder because they have to stabilize the pelvis before contracting.

Don't lift the head off the support. This makes the ab trainer less effective.

Don't pull with the arms. This makes the exercise less effective and may place stress on the neck.

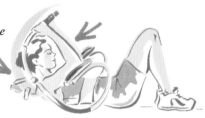

OBLIQUE CURL: *Works the internal and external obliques.*

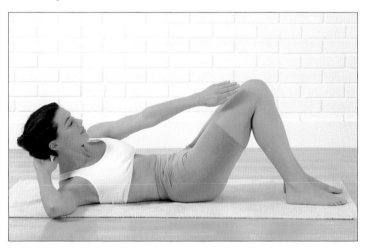

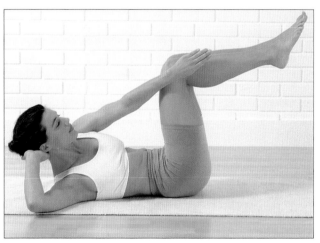

Lie flat on your back with knees bent and feet hip width apart. Exhaling, contract the abdominal muscles, and with your left arm, reach around your right knee, lifting your left shoulder slightly off the floor, until you feel a stretch in your midsection. Keep your right shoulder and lower back pressed into the floor. Hold briefly at the top position, then, inhaling, lower back to the floor.

Advanced
Perform this exercise in the same way as the oblique curl but with your knees lifted at a 90° angle and your feet parallel. Reach up past your knee toward your toes. As with the advanced crunch exercise, this makes the oblique muscles work harder.

Legs and Feet

Healthy, strong leg and foot muscles are the basis of mobility and are vital for your independence and quality of life, particularly as you age. With the increase in sedentary jobs, many people are missing out on an essential daily workout.

Although a low level of fitness may first present itself as aches in the leg muscles after unaccustomed exercise, it is relatively easy to isolate and strengthen the muscles of the legs.

The anatomy of the legs

Covering the front of the thigh is the quadriceps. Although it consists of four separate parts, the principal combined action of these parts is to straighten the knee (extension). The quadriceps also works during normal walking, especially when going down slopes or stairs, during which it contracts to provide a breaking force. After an extensive bout of unaccustomed walking on hills, it is often the quadriceps muscle that is sore the next day.

Covering the inner thigh are the adductors, which consist of a group of muscles that bring the leg to the midline (adduction).

The main buttock muscle, gluteus maximus, is the largest muscle of the body, providing much of the power for walking up stairs or rising from

COMPLEMENTARY EXERCISES FOR LEGS AND FEET

▶ Climbing stairs is especially good exercise for the legs and buttocks, but you don't have to use complicated machinery at the gym. Simply stepping up and down stairs at home or at work for 6 to 12 minutes at a time will be of benefit.

▶ Ballet has always been a rigorous workout for the feet, with extensive flexing and arching required. If you suffer from flat feet, ballet exercises may be very beneficial.

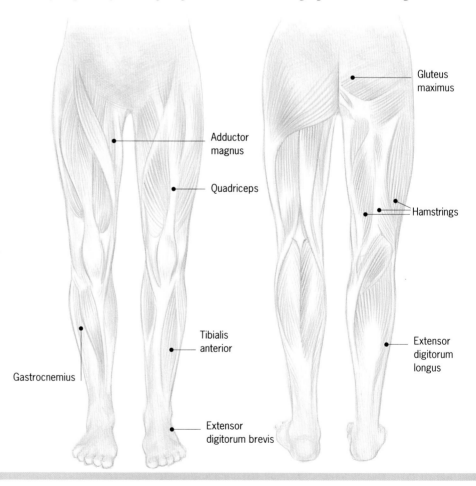

- Adductor magnus
- Quadriceps
- Gastrocnemius
- Tibialis anterior
- Extensor digitorum brevis
- Gluteus maximus
- Hamstrings
- Extensor digitorum longus

a chair. Like many muscles in this part of the body, it assists with good posture by maintaining the correct pelvic tilt.

The other main buttocks muscles, the gluteus medius and gluteus minimus, lie beneath the gluteus maximus. They act together to lift the leg out to the side (abductors). And when a person is walking, they play a key role in balancing the pelvis as one leg is lifted off the ground. Collectively, the gluteus muscles are known as the gluteals.

At the back of the upper leg are the hamstrings, which are formed from three muscles. They cross both the hip and the knee joint and can therefore assist the gluteus maximus in pulling the leg backward (hip extension) or can work to bend the knee (flexion).

The anatomy of the feet

On the front of the lower leg is the tibialis anterior and the many extensor muscles of the toes. The tibialis anterior is the largest muscle on the front of the leg. It causes the foot to lift up (dorsiflexion). The sole of the foot consists of numerous muscles and tendons that act to bend the toes and maintain the arch when you are standing or walking.

Leg and feet problems

Many women are concerned about their thighs as their major shape problem. In premenopausal women the thighs and buttocks are a major fat storage site, so any weight gain will result in fat being stored there. Toning and strengthening exercises can improve their appearance, but will not eliminate the fat.

Both men and women are affected by shortening of the leg muscles, which can cause not only tightness but also back pain. It is a common problem for people of all ages who spend long periods sitting.

Fallen arches are the most common foot problem, but regular exercise can help prevent the associated pain.

SHAPE CHALLENGE
Flat feet

The arches of the feet form gradually after birth as the supportive ligaments and muscles in the soles of the feet develop. In some people arches do not form, usually because of an inherited defect, but the condition is generally painless. However, if arches collapse in adult life, the feet often ache when a person is walking or standing, and the toe extensors on top of the foot may become tight and painful. Flat feet can be caused by a rapid increase in weight or a weakening of the muscles resulting from a neurological or muscular disease.

CASE HISTORY

Betty is 50 years old and has just returned to work after recovering from a major operation. The enforced convalescence period has led to a major weight gain, and Betty has been distressed to find that walking is now very painful. Her doctor has diagnosed fallen arches and has recommended that she wear arch supports, but he has also advised her to undertake some exercise.

Betty's regimen

▶ *Betty needs to develop with her doctor and a fitness instructor a total health and fitness program to deal with her condition. She will have to adjust her diet and do some aerobic exercise to lose some pounds because excess weight is contributing to the problem.*

▶ *Aerobic exercise will be difficult until her arches strengthen, so she will need to perform regularly some arch extension exercises to build the muscles. Slowly rolling her foot over a tennis ball for 5 minutes daily will also help.*

SHAPE CHALLENGE
Tight hamstrings

Hamstrings are probably best known as the muscles that can be painfully pulled by athletes. However, hamstrings can also be damaged more insidiously. Because they perform the function of bending the knee and swinging the leg backward from the thigh, they can become shortened by long periods of sitting and thus susceptible to injury. And because the hamstrings are attached by tendons to the pelvis, they affect the way in which the pelvis moves; when they are tight, they can cause lower back pain.

CASE HISTORY

Jonathan is a 42-year-old executive who is largely deskbound. Until a few months ago, he enjoyed going for a jog at least three times a week, but his workload has dramatically increased lately and he now doesn't find any time for exercise. At the end of the working day, Jonathan often experiences lower backache, and his leg muscles feel tight.

Jonathan's regimen

▶ *Jonathan should have his back pain checked by a doctor, but it is possible that his hamstrings have shortened from lack of activity. He must try to take regular breaks for stretching at work, sitting for no more than 45 minutes without a break. He should also check his sitting posture and try to avoid slouching in his chair.*

▶ *Jonathan could perform some leg exercises discreetly in his chair at work. However, he also needs to make regular time in his life for exercise once more.*

Exercises to target the legs and feet

Warming up and stretching are very important before doing leg and feet exercises. Because these muscles are so vital for general mobility, severe aches in them may cause you not to exercise. This is easily avoided with proper stretching and a gradual buildup in intensity.

LEG STRETCHES

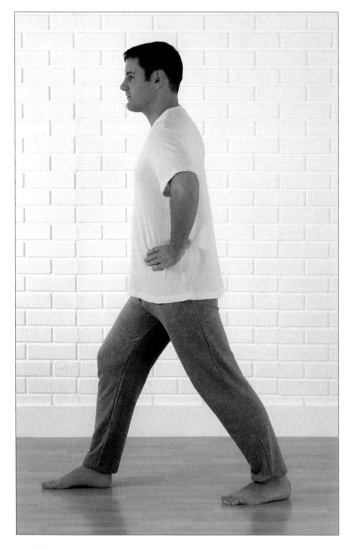

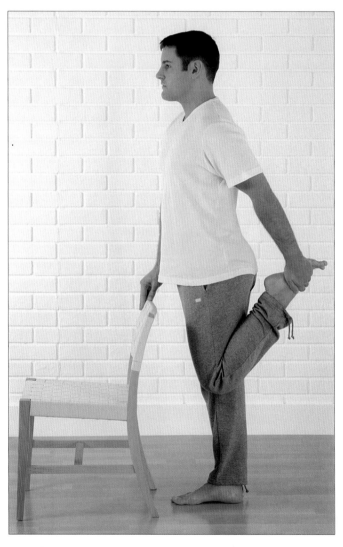

Calf stretch
Standing with your feet hip width apart and feet facing forward, take a step forward with your right leg, keeping the knee slightly bent. Press the heel of the left leg into the floor until you feel the stretch in the rear calf muscle of this leg. Hold the stretch for 20 to 30 seconds, keeping your weight centered over your hips. Step backward with your right leg to return to the starting position. Repeat with the other leg.

Quadriceps stretch
Using a chair for support, centralize your weight over your hips. Lift your left foot behind you, grasp the foot with your hand, and pull it up toward your buttocks, pressing the knee forward to keep it parallel with the supporting knee. Keeping the supporting knee slightly bent, touch your heel to your buttocks. Hold the stretch for 20 to 30 seconds. Lower the leg slowly to the floor and repeat with the other leg.

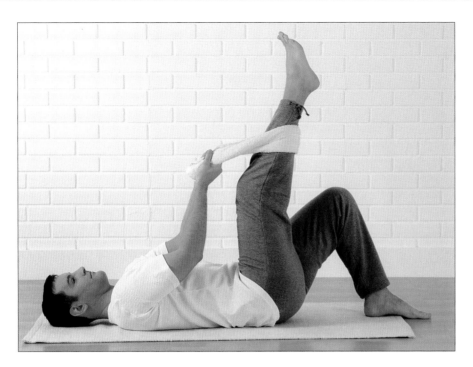

Hamstring stretch

For this stretch you will need a mat and a towel. Lie on your back with your weight evenly distributed and knees bent. Contract the abdominal muscles and press your lower back flat onto the mat. Raise one leg and loop a towel around it. Use the towel to ease the leg gently toward the upper body until you feel a stretch. Hold the stretch for 20 to 30 seconds. Lower the leg slowly and repeat with the other leg.

LUNGE: *Works quadriceps, hamstrings, and gluteals.*

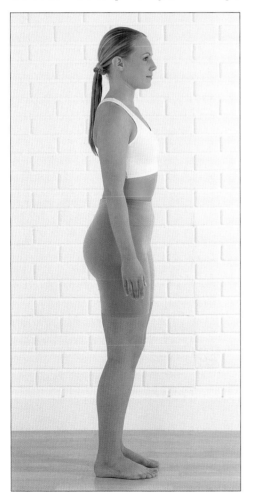

1 *Stand straight with your feet together and abdominal muscles contracted. Throughout the exercise, keep your back straight and your head in line with your spine.*

2 *Inhaling, take a giant stride forward, following with the body. (Your front knee should not go beyond your toes.) Hold the pose briefly at the bottom position, then push back to the starting position, exhaling. Repeat with other leg.*

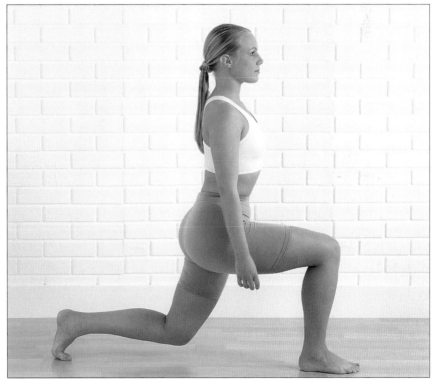

SQUAT: *Works quadriceps, hamstrings, and gluteals.*

Stand with your abdominal muscles contracted and feet hip width apart. With your arms stretched out in front of you, bend at the knees and lower the body, inhaling as you go. Keep your head in line with your spine and stop before your thighs are parallel to the floor. Hold briefly at the bottom position and then, exhaling, push up to the starting position.

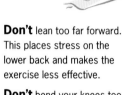

Keep the back straight.

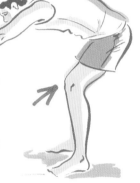

Don't lean too far forward. This places stress on the lower back and makes the exercise less effective.

Don't bend your knees too deeply.

CALF RAISE

Use a chair to aid your balance. With your body straight and abdominal muscles contracted, press up until you are on tiptoe, exhaling. Briefly hold the top position before slowly lowering to the floor, inhaling as you go.

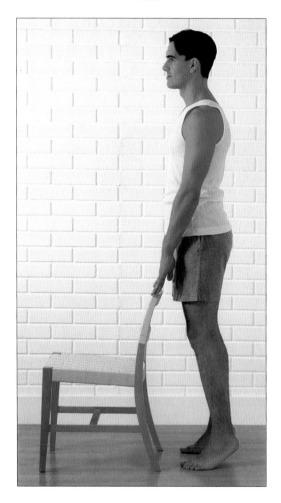

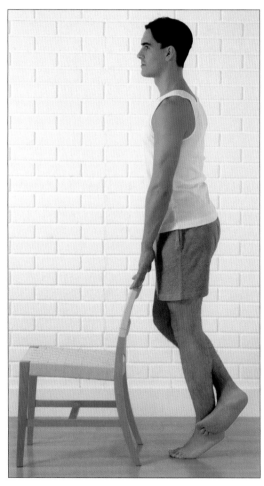

Advanced calf raise
Increase the intensity of the calf raise by performing the exercise on one foot with the other crossed behind the ankle, as shown.

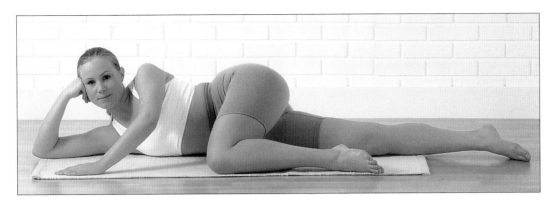

INNER THIGH RAISE:

Works adductors.

1 *Lie on one side with your body aligned and one knee bent. Support your head with one hand and your body with the other, as shown.*

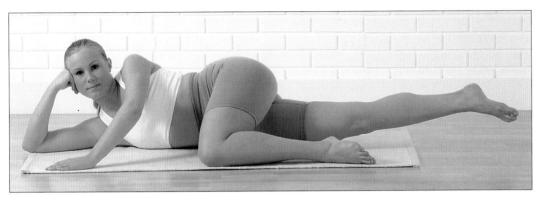

2 *With abdominal muscles contracted, slowly raise straight leg as far as is comfortable, exhaling. Take care not to lock the knee and keep your toes pointing toward the floor. Lower with control, inhaling. Keep movements slow and controlled. Repeat with the other leg.*

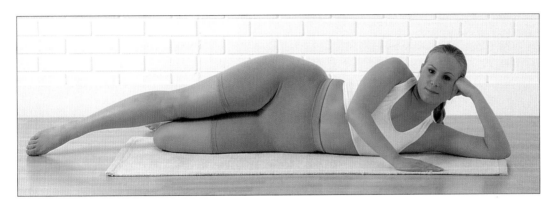

OUTER THIGH RAISE:

Works gluteals.

1 *Lie on one side with the knee that is in contact with the floor bent at a 90° angle. Support your head with one hand and your body with the other, as shown.*

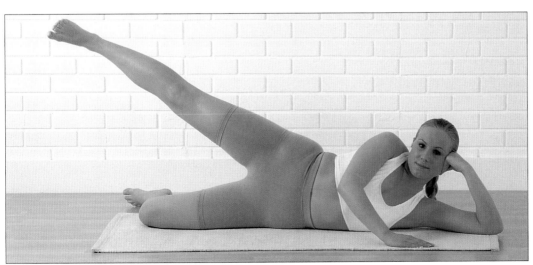

2 *With your abdominal muscles contracted, slowly raise your upper leg, exhaling as you go. Take care not to lock the knee. Lower with control, inhaling. Repeat with the other leg.*

GLUTE LIFT:

Works gluteals.

1 *You will need a mat for this exercise. Start on your hands and knees with your hands placed directly beneath your shoulders, knees slightly apart, and elbows unlocked. Looking down at the mat, contract your abdominal muscles, keeping your lower back flat. Straighten your right leg and rest on your toes.*

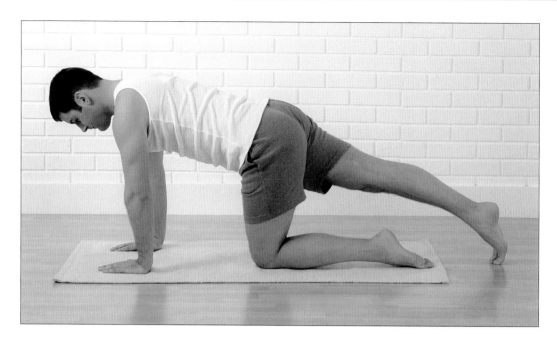

2 *Squeezing your buttock, lift your leg to a horizontal position, concentrating on contracting the buttock. Hold the contraction for 5 seconds. Perform the exercise 10 times, then repeat with the other leg.*

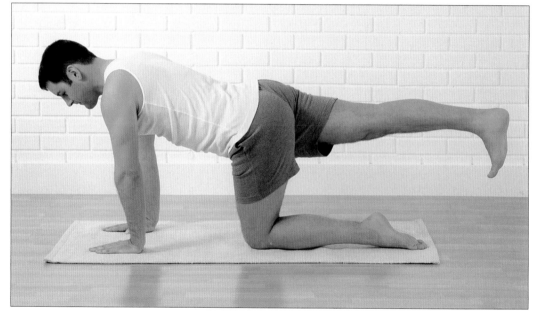

Don't tilt your head backward as this could strain your neck.

Don't relax the abdominal muscles because your back may twist and be injured.

Don't allow your arms to go beyond a 90° angle with your trunk.

Don't bend the raised leg; keep it straight with knee unlocked.

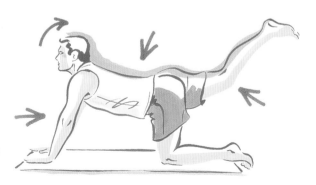

LEG PRESS:

Works quadriceps,
hamstrings, and gluteals.

Position your feet
so that the bend at
your knees is 90°.

1 Before you begin, check
the weight stack and
adjust the seat. Start with
your knees and hips at a 90°
angle to your trunk and
your feet flat on the foot
support. Keep your lower
back and head in contact
with the back support and
grip the bars, as shown.

WHEAT GERM OIL

Wheat germ oil is one of the
richest natural sources of vitamin
E, an important skin-healing
nutrient. It also contains other
vitamins and essential fatty acids
that strengthen the skin.
Although it is too rich to use on
its own, it can be very beneficial
when added in small amounts to
creams and lotions.

Keep your feet
flat against the
foot support.

2 Push your body slowly up
and away from the foot
support, exhaling. Make sure
your feet stay flat against the
support. You should feel a
stretch in the whole of your
upper leg. Hold briefly at the
top position before slowly
returning to the starting
position, inhaling. Start with
one set of 10 to 20 repetitions
for the first 4 weeks, building
to three sets by week 9.

Don't place the feet too far
down the support; this will
place stress on the knee joint.

Don't lock the knees. This not
only makes the exercise less
effective but may also damage
the knees.

Don't arch the lower back
because this may cause injury.

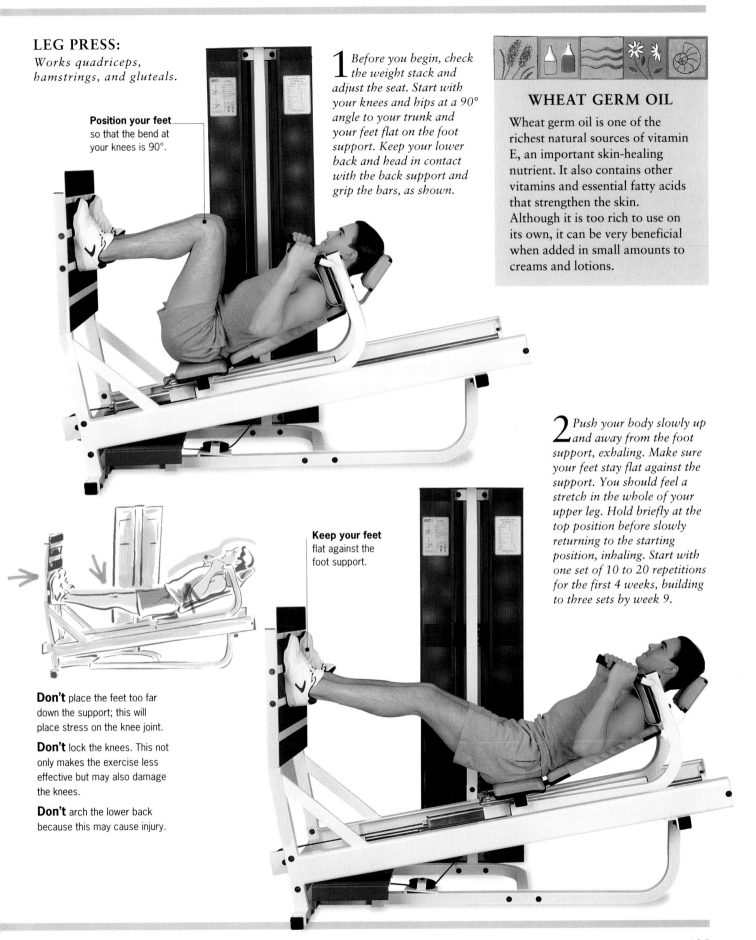

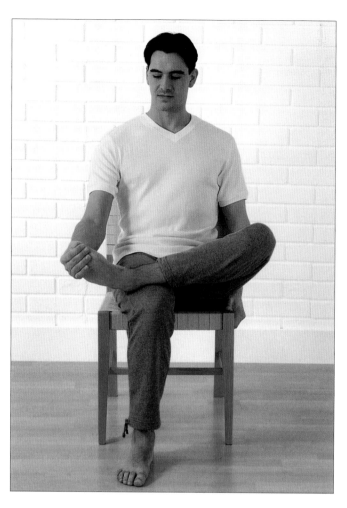

◄ TOE EXTENSORS STRETCH

Cross one leg over the other. Keeping both legs in contact at all times, grasp the foot and gently pull it toward you and upward. Hold for 10 to 30 seconds; repeat with the other foot.

ARCH EXERCISE

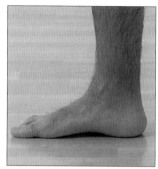

1 *This exercise will strengthen the arch of your foot and may relieve pain and tension felt as a result of fallen arches. Stand with some of your weight on one foot.*

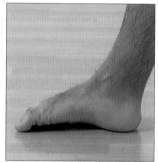

2 *Draw in your toes to arch your foot. Hold this position for 20 seconds. Now relax the foot for 20 seconds. Repeat this exercise 3 to 5 times with each foot.*

DORSI FLEXION: *Works anterior tibialis.*

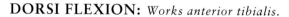

1 *Loop an elastic band around a fixed object, such as a heavy table leg. Sit with one leg straight out in front of you and your foot inserted through the band. There should be mild tension in the band at this starting position.*

2 *Pull the foot toward you and hold for 2 seconds, then slowly relax. Repeat 10 to 20 times.*

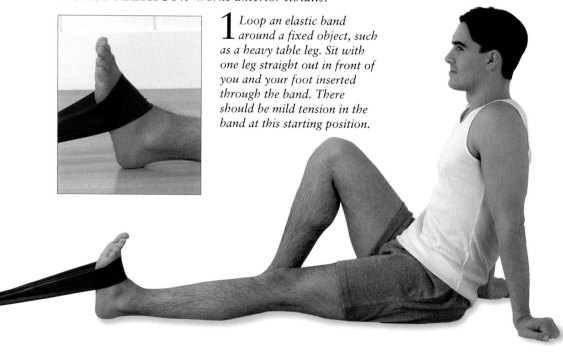

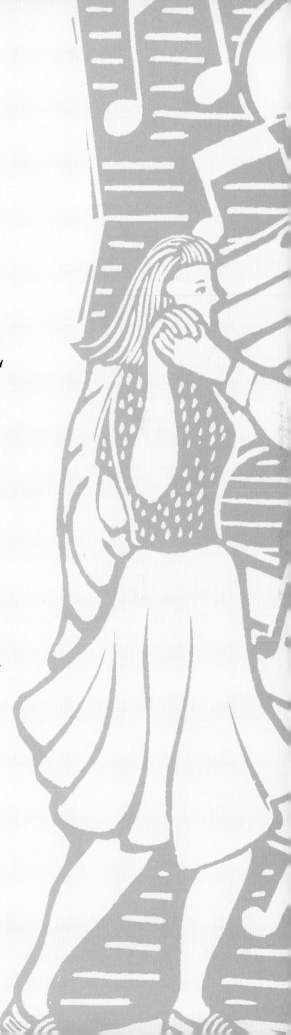

CHAPTER 6

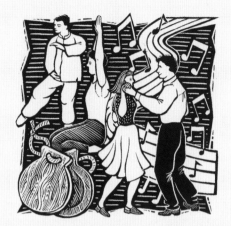

ALTERNATIVE WAYS OF SHAPING UP

There are so many exercise options to explore these days that shaping up can be a stimulating or mind-expanding experience. Many alternative approaches focus on the mind, body, and spirit as a whole, aiming not only to tone the body but also to benefit the inner self through creative expression, meditation, and relaxation.

IMPROVING BODY SHAPE WITH YOGA

The Indian art of yoga is more than just a form of physical exercise. In addition to improving strength and flexibility, yoga promotes inner calm and the health of the internal organs.

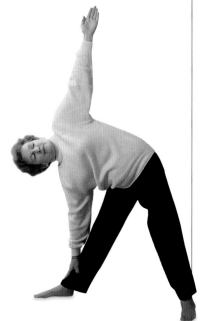

YOGA FOR FLEXIBILITY
Flexibility is one of the most important aspects of yoga. By emphasizing muscle relaxation at the beginning of a routine, even the most challenging positions become achievable.

Yoga, both an ancient philosophy and a system of exercises, has been practiced in India for over 5,000 years. It has traditionally held the unique status of being a practical part of Ayurvedic medicine (see page 42), as well as a form of spiritual devotion. However, it is not necessary to subscribe to any particular set of beliefs to practice yoga successfully; people from all cultures and walks of life can enjoy its mental and physical benefits.

From a shaping-up perspective, yoga can be quite demanding. The postures require both flexibility and a surprising degree of muscular strength and stamina. Yet anyone of any age can benefit from practicing yoga. And its special breathing techniques can ease stress and fatigue and boost energy.

HOW YOGA WORKS

There are eight fundamental principles, or sutras, on which yoga is built. The first two are *yama* and *niyama*—the moral and ethical codes that help a person to conduct a life that is disciplined and does not harm any other individual. *Asana* and *pranayama* constitute the third and fourth sutras of yoga. They require physical control and mental discipline in order for the body to be mastered and its desires tamed.

Mastery of the first four sutras leads the student to the higher, or internal, ones called *samyama* in Sanskrit. *Pratyahara*, the fifth sutra, requires withdrawal from the distractions of the outside world to focus on the soul. The sixth is *dharana*, meaning "concentration." The aim here is to focus

---

VISUALIZING YOUR CHAKRAS

According to yogic belief, seven energy centers, or chakras, span the body from the base of the spine to the head, linking the mind with the body. Each chakra is depicted as a lotus flower, has its own particular color that corresponds to one in the rainbow, and is associated with a psychological or spiritual function, such as love or survival.

MEDITATIVE FOCUS
To concentrate on the associations linked with a particular chakra, imagine it superimposed on your body, its color glowing strongly.

Crown, or *sahasrara,* chakra is related to oneness and wisdom. Color: violet.

Brow, or *ajna,* chakra is related to clarity of thought and mental agility. Color: indigo.

Throat, or *vishuddi,* chakra is related to creativity. Color: bright blue.

Heart, or *anahata,* chakra is related to feelings of love and peace. Color: green.

Solar plexus, or *manipura,* chakra is related to power and will. Color: yellow.

Sacral, or *svadisthana,* chakra is related to sexuality and pleasure. Color: orange.

Base, or *muladhara,* chakra is related to survival and grounding. Color: red.

Warming up for

Yoga and T'ai Chi

Both yoga and t'ai chi promote mental focus and physical flexibility. To prepare for a session, it is important not only to stretch and warm up all the major muscle groups of the body but also to calm and focus the mind with meditation.

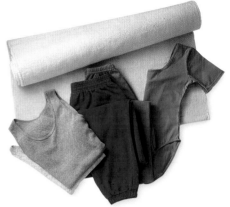

Start your yoga preparation with a period of meditation to calm and prepare your mind. Begin by sitting in a comfortable upright position (a crossed-leg position on the floor is typical) with shoulders relaxed. Close your eyes and concentrate on breathing slowly and rhythmically, without force. Counting your breaths can help divert your mind from external thoughts. Count in sets of five inhaled breaths, focusing on the physical sensation of the breath in the nostrils as it enters the body.

EXERCISE ESSENTIALS
Wear comfortable exercise clothing in breathable fabrics. A mat or towel is useful for yoga floor work.

STRETCHES TO WARM UP YOUR MUSCLES

After about 10 minutes of meditation, you can move on to a physical warmup. It is important to enter into yoga gradually, so always begin with a series of exercises and stretches that increase the mobility of the joints and warm and stretch the muscles. The warmup will help to release any tension stored in the body, allowing a fuller range of movement during the rest of the session. This reduces the risk of injury and will enable you to benefit fully from your yoga session.

Combine the stretches shown here with those featured on pages 94–136 to create a warmup that begins at the top of your head and works down toward your feet. As you do these stretches, tension will drop away.

Try to stretch to the same point when you repeat the stretch on the other side.

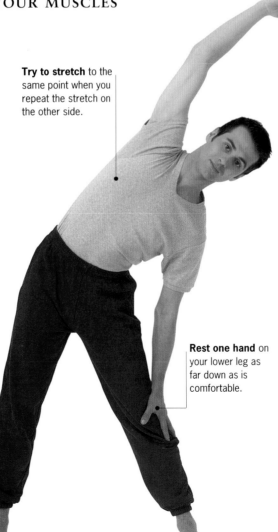

Rest one hand on your lower leg as far down as is comfortable.

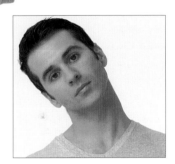

NECK STRETCH
Tilt your head slowly toward your right shoulder, then slowly return it to the center and tilt it to the left. Repeat the exercise five times.

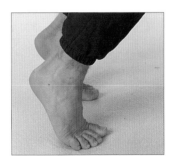

FOOT FLEXOR
Holding onto the back of a chair for support and bending your knees slightly, slowly lift heels off the floor, then lower them. Repeat four times.

SIDE STRETCH
Stand with your feet wide apart. Slide your left hand down your left leg and extend your right arm over your head to the left as far as you can, following with your upper body. Do not lean forward. Hold the stretch for 10 to 20 seconds, then slowly return to the starting position. Repeat the stretch on the other side.

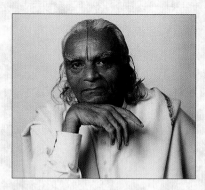

Origins

Born in India in 1918, B.K.S. Iyengar has devoted his life to the practice of yoga and has been honored by the Indian government for his efforts. He has systematized more than 2,000 postures and breathing techniques, developed props to assist in poses, and worked extensively on adapting many postures to make them more accessible and beneficial to people with disabilities.

PRESENT-DAY GURU
B.K.S. Iyengar, a renowned authority on yoga, has greatly influenced how Westerners practice it.

the mind in order to prevent it from wandering or becoming distracted. This leads to the seventh sutra, called *dhayana* or meditation. The final sutra that can be achieved is the trance state, *samadhi*, which is the state of heightened consciousness that can lead to ultimate mental freedom.

Over the centuries many different schools of yoga have developed, each placing a different emphasis on the various aspects of yogic practice. One of the most popular forms in the West and an easily accessible form for the novice is hatha yoga. The Sanskrit word *hatha* can be broken into two elements: *ha,* meaning "sun," and *tha,* meaning "moon." This pairing of opposites represents the yogic ideal of balance between the mind and body and between active energy and passive relaxation. When neither of these aspects outweighs the other, we perform better in our day-to-day lives and experience optimum levels of health.

Hatha yoga takes the physical body as a starting point, emphasizing posture (asanas) and breathing (pranayama) as a means of achieving health. A practical system of concentration and mental discipline is used to bring the body into various postures that strengthen the muscles, correct misalignments of the back and limbs, massage the internal organs, and encourage a state of relaxation and emotional tranquillity.

BASIC YOGA MOVEMENTS

Yoga exercises involve a variety of postures and positions, done while standing, sitting, lying down, or kneeling. The following exercises offer a sample of some of the many postures, or asanas, that can improve your flexibility, muscle tone, and balance.

RISHI'S POSTURE

1 Begin by standing with your feet together. Transfer your weight to your left leg and bend your right leg at the knee without moving the position of your thigh. Take hold of your right foot with your right hand and draw it up toward your buttocks.

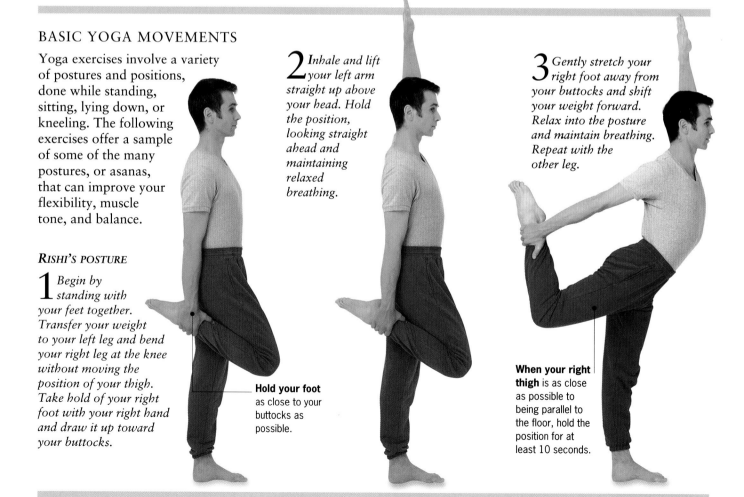

2 Inhale and lift your left arm straight up above your head. Hold the position, looking straight ahead and maintaining relaxed breathing.

Hold your foot as close to your buttocks as possible.

3 Gently stretch your right foot away from your buttocks and shift your weight forward. Relax into the posture and maintain breathing. Repeat with the other leg.

When your right thigh is as close as possible to being parallel to the floor, hold the position for at least 10 seconds.

DID YOU KNOW?

According to Indian mythology, the Hindu sage Patanjali founded the practice of yoga in order to give mankind spiritual harmony and serenity. He also gave humans articulate speech through the invention of grammar and bodily health through his innovations in medicine. He is depicted in Indian iconography as half serpent and half human in form.

How yoga improves flexibility and tone

A yoga routine often begins with breathing exercises called pranayama. By focusing intently on the breath, extraneous thoughts and anxieties are screened out and the mind is better connected with the body, allowing the participant to access his or her potential life energy, or *prana*.

Pranayama strengthens the respiratory muscles, calms the nervous system, and relaxes the body in order to prepare it for the asanas. Good breath control, essential to maintain stable postures during a yoga routine, can be very effective in helping to cope with stressful situations as well. One approach is to visualize the body drawing in life energy with each inhalation and expelling waste products and toxins with each exhalation, breathing them onto a fire that burns them away. Combining breath control with the various yoga postures revitalizes both the body and mind.

Asanas are the physical expression of, as well as the practical route to, achieving the unification of body and spirit, which is the aim of all forms of yoga. Asanas are stretching postures performed without force in a slow, relaxed manner. They are designed to release tension from the joints, muscles, ligaments, and tendons, as well as to tone up the internal systems of the body.

Although the movements in most forms of yoga are nonvigorous and slow, they still provide a thorough muscular workout that improves tone, strength, and flexibility. The stretches are static and held for a longer

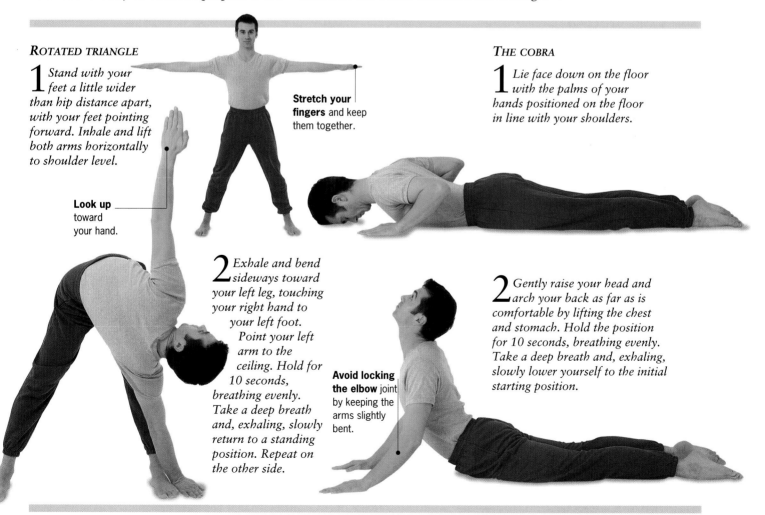

ROTATED TRIANGLE

1 *Stand with your feet a little wider than hip distance apart, with your feet pointing forward. Inhale and lift both arms horizontally to shoulder level.*

Stretch your fingers and keep them together.

Look up toward your hand.

2 *Exhale and bend sideways toward your left leg, touching your right hand to your left foot. Point your left arm to the ceiling. Hold for 10 seconds, breathing evenly. Take a deep breath and, exhaling, slowly return to a standing position. Repeat on the other side.*

THE COBRA

1 *Lie face down on the floor with the palms of your hands positioned on the floor in line with your shoulders.*

2 *Gently raise your head and arch your back as far as is comfortable by lifting the chest and stomach. Hold the position for 10 seconds, breathing evenly. Take a deep breath and, exhaling, slowly lower yourself to the initial starting position.*

Avoid locking the elbow joint by keeping the arms slightly bent.

Balanced breath

The yogic breathing technique of inhaling through one nostril and exhaling through the other is believed to unite the opposing sides of our nature and eliminate imbalance between them. The right nostril is associated with activity and rationality, the left nostril with our passive emotional side. In Ayurvedic medicine this technique is used as a means of balancing the doshas (see page 46).

period than the stretches in other forms of exercise. Ideally, an asana is held for at least 20 to 30 seconds, although it may take some practice to achieve this length of time. When a muscle is held long enough in the stretch, it relaxes and increases slightly in length. The regular practice of asanas over time leads to a longer, leaner musculature, as well as the increased muscle tone and strength typically achieved with other forms of exercise. While one muscle is stretching, another has to remain contracted in order to maintain steady posture. This static contraction also helps to develop physical strength and endurance without putting stress on the joints and skeleton.

Maneuvering into and out of each position smoothly can be difficult at first. But as the exercises become more familiar, communication between mind and body also improves, resulting in better flow of movement, balance, and coordination.

If a joint gets slightly out of position and is not subsequently realigned properly, the muscles and tendons

around it become tense and knotted as the body attempts to stabilize the problem area. This results in stiffness and pain. Practicing asanas can correct misalignments, freeing up movement. The concentrated training that both muscles and joints receive also contributes to increased flexibility.

You should learn yoga in a class, where a teacher can help you not only to attain the correct positions for the postures and do them in a sequence that keeps the body in balance but also to understand the philosophy behind yogic practice. Once you are familiar with several routines, you can practice on your own or with a tape.

If you are practicing at home, try to choose a time when there will be no distractions. It is important not to practice yoga on a full stomach, so first thing in the morning is ideal. Otherwise, allow plenty of time between a meal and the start of your session. Wear comfortable and loose-fitting clothing so you can move freely. You do not need special equipment to practice yoga, but a mat can be helpful for some postures.

ENDING A SESSION

To finish a yoga session, choose positions that gently stretch the muscles and can be held for a while to allow body and mind to completely relax. The child pose not only has a calming effect but also increases flexibility in the hips, while the corpse pose is so relaxing it can induce sleep.

THE CHILD POSE

1 Kneel, sitting on your heels. Keeping your back straight, stretch your body upward. Link your fingers with palms facing forward and raise your arms above your head. Release your fingers, keeping the palms facing forward.

Relax your arms by your sides with palms facing upward.

2 Bring your arms down by your sides. Take a deep breath and, exhaling, slowly fold your body down over your legs until your forehead is gently touching the floor. Hold the position for about a minute, then take another deep breath and, exhaling, slowly return to the starting position.

Allow your feet to fall gently outward.

Your arms should be held at about 45° to your body.

THE CORPSE POSE

This position can be held for 5 minutes at the start and end of a session and can also be practiced as a relaxation technique between the more difficult postures of a yoga session. Lie flat on your back with your arms and legs apart. Close your eyes and lie still. Relax your body and feel the contact of your back with the floor. Breathe evenly.

TONING UP WITH T'AI CHI

The slow, controlled movements of t'ai chi have been practiced for centuries by the Chinese as a way of exercising the body and focusing the mind to promote health and longevity.

T'ai chi is formally classed as a martial art but is practiced today mainly for its beneficial effect on emotional and physical well-being. Sometimes described as an "internal martial art," it differs from other Eastern martial arts forms, such as judo and aikido, in that it is mainly non-combative and uses internal techniques, such as breath control, visualization, and channeling of energy, to achieve psychologi-cal and physical strength. Although other martial arts are also good for toning up and developing muscular strength, balance, stamina, and speed of reaction, t'ai chi has a greater focus on spiritual aspects.

THE HISTORY OF T'AI CHI
According to tradition, the 13th-century Taoist priest Zhang San Feng created t'ai chi after witnessing a fight between a crane

BASIC T'AI CHI MOVEMENTS

The movements of t'ai chi are slow, continuous, and purposeful, working through a designated series of flowing forms or postures, which together create what is called a set. Start each posture by standing with the feet slightly wider than hip distance apart. Bend the knees a little and focus on your back to maintain an upright, centered position that feels natural to the spine. The aim is to perform each stance with strength and power in the legs while keeping the shoulders relaxed and free from tension.

SINGLE WHIP

1 *Put your weight on your left leg and keep your right leg slightly bent and soft. Make the shape of a bird's beak with your right hand and place the fingers of the left hand lightly on the right wrist.*

2 *Take a wide step back with your right leg and shift your weight forward, bending your left knee. Stretch your left arm forward with the fingers pointing up and pull the right arm back with the fingers pointing down in the bird's beak position.*

Keep your back straight but not tensed.

Keep the bent knee soft, not locked.

and a snake. Surprised to see that the bird's calm and graceful defensive movements proved a strong match for the explosive strikes of the snake, he was inspired to develop a martial art that took as its philosophy the idea of using minimum force to combat maximum strength. Since its foundation was established, t'ai chi has evolved into many different styles, some emphasizing combat and others completely given over to improving health.

The full name of the art, t'ai chi chuan, comes from the Chinese *t'ai chi*, meaning "cosmos," and *chuan fa*, meaning "way of the fist," revealing its roots as a fighting style. However, one of the most popular forms practiced today is the Yang style developed by Yang Deng Fu (1883–1936), who eliminated many of the more aggressive movements, such as jumps, kicks, and straight punches, in order to emphasize the health aspect of t'ai chi chuan. Because of this move away from the martial aspect, many practitioners drop the reference to combat and simply call this style t'ai chi.

DID YOU KNOW?

The relaxing effect of t'ai chi on the mind and its beneficial effects on physical health have prompted insurance companies in Germany to pay their clients greater dividends if they learn t'ai chi or chi kung, a related martial art.

How t'ai chi works

The graceful and controlled movements of t'ai chi help to stimulate the flow of energy (*chi*) around the body along the channels also used in acupuncture. Regular practice replenishes lost energy, improving both your mental and physical shape.

In traditional Chinese medicine the energy system is considered the basic foundation of health upon which all other bodily systems are built. If our energy is blocked, we become ill. T'ai chi clears energy blockages, thus helping to prevent serious illnesses, such as hypertension, asthma, and rheumatism. T'ai chi is now widely recognized as a

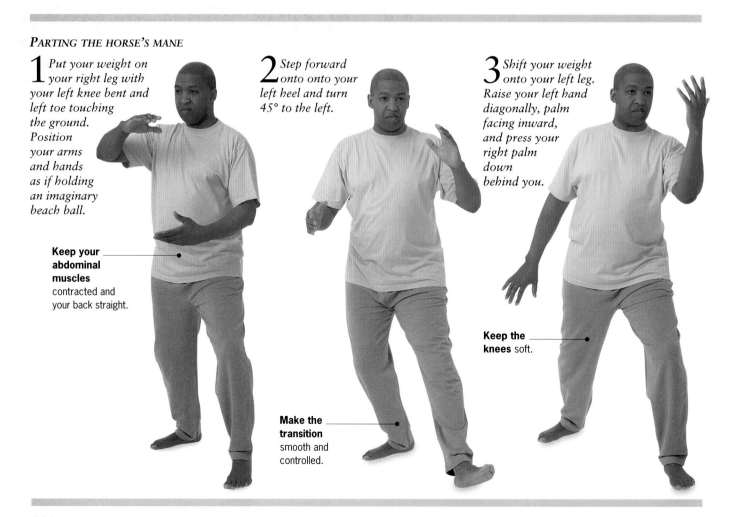

PARTING THE HORSE'S MANE

1 *Put your weight on your right leg with your left knee bent and left toe touching the ground. Position your arms and hands as if holding an imaginary beach ball.*

Keep your abdominal muscles contracted and your back straight.

2 *Step forward onto onto your left heel and turn 45° to the left.*

Make the transition smooth and controlled.

3 *Shift your weight onto your left leg. Raise your left hand diagonally, palm facing inward, and press your right palm down behind you.*

Keep the knees soft.

therapy for reducing stress and increasing mobility in the elderly. Some believe it may even be helpful in the prevention of cancer.

The concept of yin and yang is an important part of t'ai chi. The two words signify opposing pairs of forces—for example, masculine and feminine, light and dark—that govern the universe. Imbalance between these forces results in physical or emotional illness. T'ai chi restores balance through movements that alternate between hard (the yang, or masculine, principle) and soft (the yin, or feminine, principle) to promote calm, mental clarity, and equilibrium.

How t'ai chi improves muscle tone

Each position in t'ai chi is achieved through smooth, linking movements that may look effortless but require great control. These actions develop muscular strength in the legs as they balance, bend, straighten, and change direction or height. The slow pace of movement accentuates the effect of the exercise, and a lot of leg power is needed to hold the deep stances required. Other physical benefits include increased mobility of the spine and flexibility in the joints. If practiced correctly, t'ai chi can also prevent or relieve knee injury, which studies have shown to be the most common and disabling form of joint problems.

T'ai chi benefits the body as a whole, not only toning the muscles that are visible to the eye but also benefiting internal muscles and organs. Breath control exercises slow respiration and maximize the energy derived from breathing. T'ai chi also improves the function of the digestive system, maximizing the energy we obtain from a minimum amount of food. Food is converted into energy rather than mass, benefiting those who wish to lose excess weight.

As with any form of exercise, it is important to have a warmup, or preparation, period before a t'ai chi session. This should include gentle movements that loosen the joints and warm and stretch the muscles. Of equal importance, however, are breathing and concentration exercises to focus the mind and aid relaxation.

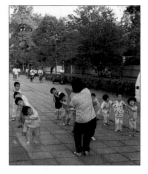

STARTING YOUNG
Regular exercise is an integral part of Chinese life from an early age. Because the movements are slow and deliberate, t'ai chi is suitable for all ages, from childhood, when it encourages development of balance and coordination, to old age, when it helps maintain joint mobility and clarity of mind.

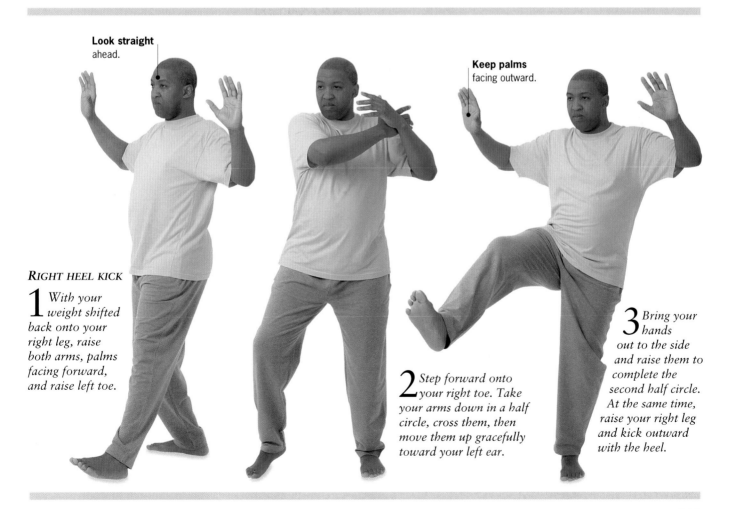

Look straight ahead.

Keep palms facing outward.

RIGHT HEEL KICK

1 *With your weight shifted back onto your right leg, raise both arms, palms facing forward, and raise left toe.*

2 *Step forward onto your right toe. Take your arms down in a half circle, cross them, then move them up gracefully toward your left ear.*

3 *Bring your hands out to the side and raise them to complete the second half circle. At the same time, raise your right leg and kick outward with the heel.*

DANCING TO GET IN SHAPE

Dancing is an instinctive movement. It provides an opportunity to explore the body's creative potential; exercise the muscles, joints, and respiratory system; and focus the mind.

Dance is our primary form of physical expression, allowing the body, mind, and spirit to work together creatively. It can be a highly disciplined, technical art or simply enjoyed as a free-flowing activity and a great way to get in shape. With so many types of dance to choose from, people, regardless of age, can find one that suits them and their personal needs. Different forms of dance offer a variety of shaping-up benefits; one style may be particularly beneficial for toning the legs or the waist, whereas another may strengthen the lower back or stomach.

BALLET
Ballet originated in the royal courts of France and Italy during the 16th century, developing out of the spectacular performances that had entertained the ruling

BASIC BALLET MOVEMENTS

Ballet offers wonderful physical benefits, no matter what your fitness level. The following exercises, based on classical ballet movements, can help you to strengthen your muscles and acquire a more graceful posture.

PLIÉ SIDE STRETCH

This exercise gently warms up the body and is particularly good for toning the inner thighs and improving balance. Regular practice improves posture by preventing slouching and relieving tension in the lower back.

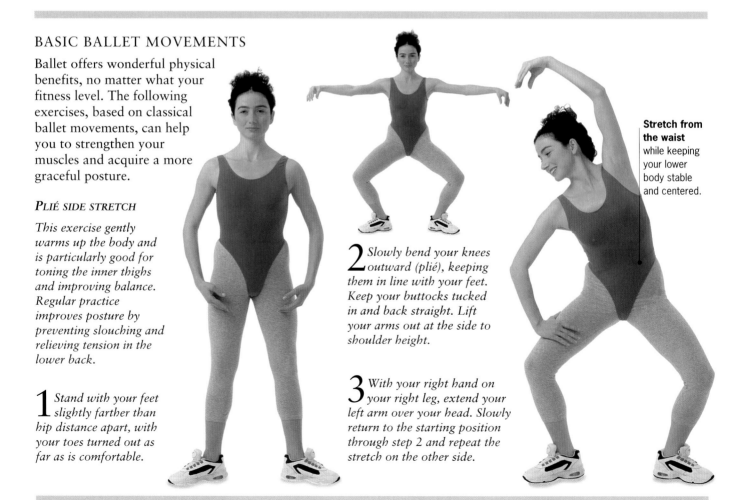

Stretch from the waist while keeping your lower body stable and centered.

1 *Stand with your feet slightly farther than hip distance apart, with your toes turned out as far as is comfortable.*

2 *Slowly bend your knees outward (plié), keeping them in line with your feet. Keep your buttocks tucked in and back straight. Lift your arms out at the side to shoulder height.*

3 *With your right hand on your right leg, extend your left arm over your head. Slowly return to the starting position through step 2 and repeat the stretch on the other side.*

classes since the Middle Ages. The steps were derived from the social dances of the time and emphasized restraint and decorum in contrast to the athleticism of modern ballet technique. During the 17th century the emphasis began to shift, and dance came to be regarded as an increasingly serious form of art, with set steps and gestures that had to be performed correctly.

Improving flexibility and tone

Ballet, which can be used to tone various areas of the body, should be performed in a smooth, controlled manner, without jerking. A warmup before starting is essential. The typical clothing for ballet practice consists of tights and a leotard. It is probably worth investing in ballet slippers, although you may dance barefoot.

Ballet can be taken to the perfection of the professional dancer or enjoyed simply as a way to improve health and fitness. The many different moods and emotions that can be expressed through ballet suit many different personalities and levels of fitness.

Origins

Classical ballet owes much to composer Jean-Baptiste Lully (1632–1687). He first emerged as a young violinist in the court band of the Sun King, Louis XIV and soon held the royal appointments of composer to the king and music master to the royal family. Lully established many of ballet's enduring traditions, including the use of women dancers, and composed music that did much to popularize the dance form.

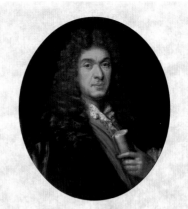

THE KING'S COMPOSER
A favorite of Louis XIV, Jean-Baptiste Lully wrote music specifically to accompany ballet.

Ballet is a highly effective way of improving overall flexibility and muscle tone; it can also help you develop coordination and balance and will do much to improve posture. Practicing ballet requires the muscles to

continued on page 150

HIP ROTATIONS

This exercise improves posture by stabilizing the pelvis and increasing flexibility in the hips; it also helps to strengthen and tone the outer thighs.

Keep your body in a straight line to protect the lower back.

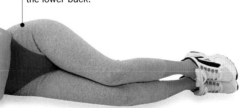

1 *Lie on your right side with your legs together. Rest your head on your right* arm and place your left arm in front of your torso to stabilize your body.

Pull in abdominal muscles to stabilize your pelvis.

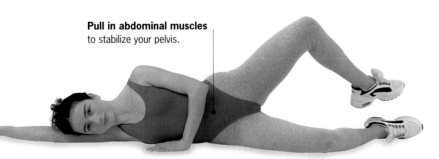

2 *Raise your left leg in a parallel position. Next, rotate the leg from the hip so that your knee is pointing toward the ceiling and your toe is* pointing down. Repeat 10 times and then turn onto your opposite side and do the exercise with the other leg.

Return to the starting position very slowly.

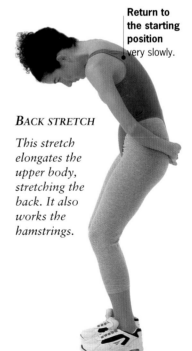

BACK STRETCH

This stretch elongates the upper body, stretching the back. It also works the hamstrings.

Stand tall to start, with your feet hip width apart. Clasp your hands behind your back and, with a slight bend at the knees, round your back forward. Gently straighten up.

The Ballet Teacher

Ballet is more accessible than many people think and is a good way to get fit and have fun at the same time. Dance classes are available for all ages and cater to people at all levels of ability, from beginners to those with a background in dance.

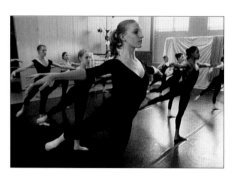

CLASS ACT
Learning ballet in a class provides a framework for self-expression, physical discipline, an elegant posture, and graceful movements.

BALLET FOR EVERYONE
Your peak flexibility occurs at around 10 years of age, but it is never too late to start ballet lessons. Dance can help to improve your self-image and confidence.

A ballet teacher provides technical supervision and stylistic guidance while safeguarding students from physical injury. A positive rapport with a teacher can also help students learn to interpret their emotions through movement.

What qualifications does a ballet teacher have?

Most ballet teachers have studied and performed with a ballet company; the ones who teach professionals usually have starred with a company of some renown. Important criteria for a good teacher include the ability to relate well to students and correct their form, to properly demonstrate movements, and to pace a class well according to students' abilities.

Who can participate?

Ballet is suitable for all ages and abilities; it is not necessary to have danced since you were a child, have a sylphlike figure, or be superfit. The pleasure of dancing and creating positive energy through a sequence of steps can be achieved at any level of ability. Don't worry if you find the steps difficult at first; do only what you are capable of without forcing your body, and you will find that your flexibility and strength gradually increase.

Are there any contraindications?

If you are pregnant or have high blood pressure, a balance disorder, or a joint complaint like arthritis, you should check with your doctor about whether ballet is an appropriate exercise for you. It can actually be beneficial for certain conditions; for example, children suffering from scoliosis can sometimes avoid permanent curvature of the spine through taking ballet lessons.

Although very young children can benefit from ballet lessons, there is debate about the age at which a girl should be allowed to go on pointe. Some professionals advise that wearing toe shoes before age 10 can be very damaging to the feet.

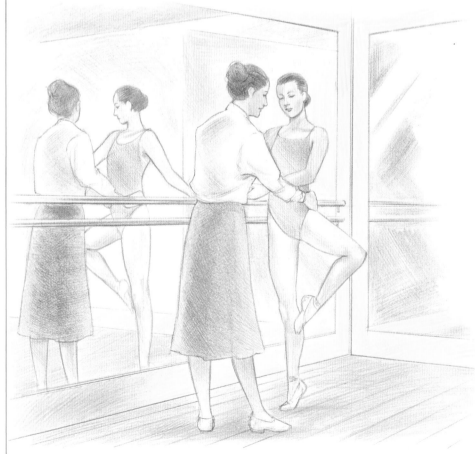

What should I expect from a dance class?

Classes are widely available for all levels of proficiency, often classified as beginning, intermediate, and advanced. However, many classes are of a general standard, and the teacher will adapt to the needs of the enrollees and offer relevant alternatives for individuals of different abilities within the group.

Ballet classes, like most forms of exercise, will always include a warmup section; this readies you for activity by getting the blood circulating to all the systems of the body, especially the major muscle groups and joints. In ballet the warmup always includes a sequence of exercises performed at the barre, which help to mobilize the joints, build strength in the muscles, and provide the groundwork for the more dynamic floor exercises.

Floor exercises, which comprise the main part of a ballet class, are usually divided into sections— graceful and slow arm movements (*port de bras*); technique work for the legs and arms; more dynamic jumps (*allegro*); turns (*pirouette*); and large jump sequences (*grande allegro*). Movements from these sections are then used to create a short routine.

A cooling-down period at the end of class is as important as the warmup. Stretching exercises are repeated, and you may be asked to hold positions for a few moments more than at the beginning of the session or to extend the leg a little farther; this is because the muscles will have greater flexibility and strength after they have been thoroughly exercised. After the stretches your heart rate and breathing should slow again.

The teacher will lead by demonstrating each movement carefully before the class performs it. He or she will also offer individual guidance to students throughout the class to ensure that posture is correct and the right groups of muscles are being worked.

What are some of the benefits of ballet?

Ballet can be appreciated at many levels, whether you participate in a professional troupe or simply enjoy dancing around the house to your favorite piece of music.

On a physical level, ballet offers excellent cardiovascular training; if the exercises are performed regularly, they can significantly improve the health of the heart and lungs. The disciplined technique of ballet also improves coordination and balance and develops muscular strength, flexibility, and endurance. All of these benefits will result in a well-defined physique, good posture, and a graceful way of moving.

Exercising the body in a creative way can achieve very positive results for your emotional well-being too. Ballet is a great way to express emotions, especially sadnesss or grief that may have been suppressed but also feelings of elation and joy.

Dancing can be a release from the inflexibility of everyday routines and an opportunity for you to become more aware of your body and explore the way it can move. Although set steps form the basis of any form of dance, they can be individually interpreted, providing a therapeutic outlet for emotional expression that can ultimately improve self-confidence and lead to a more outgoing personality.

WHAT YOU CAN DO AT HOME

You can translate the benefits of ballet from the class into every aspect of your life and use the heightened bodily awareness that ballet brings to make adjustments to your posture in everyday situations. Make a point of stopping at various intervals during your day and try

the exercises shown below. Remember that strong abdominal muscles and a strong back help to support the whole body and keep the center of balance stable. Once you achieve this status, pressure on the lower back will be relieved, which is especially important if you are sedentary for much of the day.

BACK STRETCH
From the standing position, bend your knees and fold forward from your waist, keeping your back and neck as straight as possible. You should feel your lower back releasing.

POSTURE PROMOTION
Pull yourself up to your full height. Imagine that a piece of string goes from the center point on the top of your head right down through the center of your body and that this string is pulling and lifting you upward. Make sure your shoulders are not raised or tense and think about your back and abdomen.

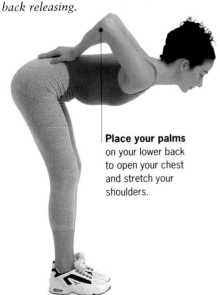

Place your palms on your lower back to open your chest and stretch your shoulders.

hold, or fixate, the body to maintain a required position, which strengthens the muscles. Simply by standing in a correct ballet posture, you statically contract your muscles. For example, the posture called "first position" tones your leg muscles by turning them out from the hips down.

Dancing a sequence of ballet steps requires a great deal of muscle work in both the lower and upper body. To bend, straighten, lift, turn, extend, and contract involves an enormous amount of physical work. However, it is important in ballet that the body remain light and the movements appear effortless and airy.

Ballet is made up of a great range of movements. Some are graceful and lyrical sequences that require tremendous muscle control to maintain balance, while others are quick and explosive. Constant practice of these sequences trains the muscles to work at various speeds, improving reaction time and coordination. At the same time, the slow, static stretching exercises that form an important part of a ballet workout develop flexibility in the muscles and increase the range of movement in the joints, allowing the body to extend to its full capability.

Although most people generally know what correct posture is, they are usually unaware of how they hold their own bodies day in and day out unless they are consciously thinking about it. This can result in habitual stooping, slouching, or rounding of the shoulders. Classically trained dancers hold an upright stance—with their shoulders back and down and stomach in—at all times. They do this effortlessly because their bodies remember to do so. Ballet exercises sensitize this physical memory, making the body more responsive and helping people to become aware of their posture in everyday life. In general, ballet strengthens muscles without building excess bulk and is wonderful for producing lean lines, agility, and a graceful carriage.

BASIC SALSA MOVEMENTS

Salsa is ideal for a couple who wants to exercise together and likes to dance. We show a few basic steps here, but you will probably have to join a class to get a real feel for the dance. It offers a good cardiovascular workout for both partners, with the woman's hips and abdomen working extra hard when turning.

1 *The starting position for all steps is to stand close together with backs straight. The man places his right arm around the woman's waist, and the woman's right hand rests lightly in the man's left hand.*

2 *Both partners bend their knees slightly. The woman steps back with her left foot and the man steps back with his right foot.*

3 *The couple steps back into the starting position, still standing close together, with the man's arm remaining around the woman's back.*

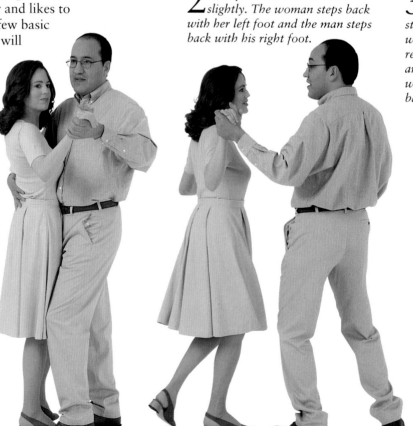
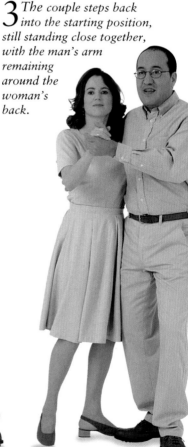

SALSA

Based on the old Cuban rhythm known as *son*, the salsa rhythm was invented by Caribbean (mainly Cuban) musicians in New York in the 1960s and 1970s. It is danced by a couple, and the man leads the woman in a tight, smooth, sensuous progression of turns, which can include more spectacular arm-spinning and multiturn figures. The soles of the feet remain close to the ground, and the knees are often slightly bent. The grace of the dance is in the movement of the hips.

Salsa for fitness

The muscles used for salsa are mainly those of the thighs and hips, so it is an exceptionally good exercise for the legs. The waistline also benefits from the constant twisting of the hips. The overall speed of movement and the fast tempo of the music make salsa an excellent form of aerobic exercise as well. In recent years the popularity of salsa has soared as people have discovered what a wonderful social activity it is. Classes are readily available in most large cities and many smaller ones, and though the more advanced steps can be quite complex and intricate, most people find the basic steps quick and easy to learn. Once you have mastered a few movements, you should be able to find nightclubs and dance events where you can practice your new skills.

FLAMENCO

Flamenco had its beginnings in Andalusia, a region of southern Spain. This area has long been a cultural melting pot, with music and dance influenced by many groups of people who settled there. It was in this atmosphere of cultural diversity toward the end of the 18th century that a local gypsy (*gitano*) form of folk music and dance called flamenco rose to prominence; it now enjoys popularity not only throughout Spain but also in many other parts of the world.

4 To prepare for turning, the man steps back with his right foot and the woman with her left, steadying herself for the turn. The man's left hand prepares to lead the woman through the turn.

5 The man remains in place and lifts his hand up, while the woman turns clockwise on her right foot. This move can be followed with another turn or a return to the starting position.

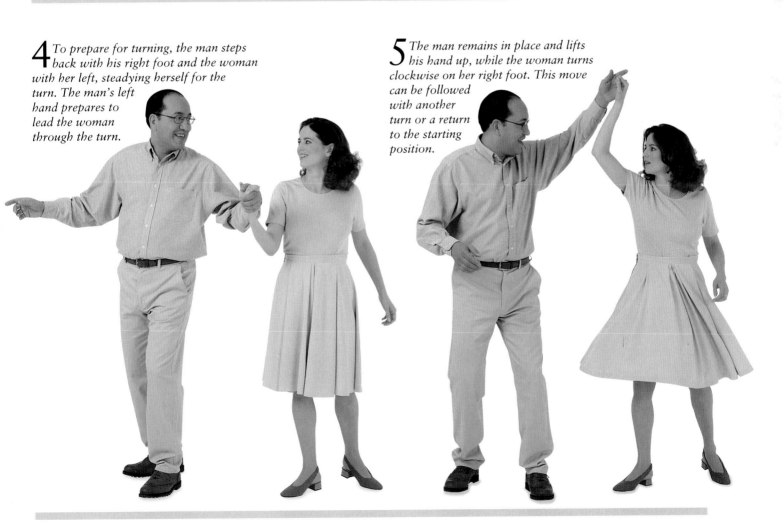

In flamenco the language of the body is concerned with the expression of intense emotions and fundamental forces that govern our lives, such as love, hate, death, fate, and morality. The communication of these feelings evokes powerful reactions in all the performers—singers, dancers, and musicians—as well as the audience.

Flamenco classes offer a space in which people are able to express their emotions freely through the passionate movements of the dance. This is in keeping with the traditional context of flamenco, which is quite intimate and not essentially about performing before a large audience.

In Spain flamenco performances are often spontaneous, taking place at a family gathering or in a tavern, with members of the gathering simply taking turns to sing, play an instrument, or dance. The audience is thus intended to participate and share in the experience, not critically observe. This intimacy differentiates flamenco from many other forms of dance. It is not an extrovert performance involving expansive spaces or spectacular acrobatic moves.

There are no age boundaries for taking up flamenco. More important than a youthful physique are maturity and experience of the joys and pains that life brings, which can usually be acquired only with age. For this reason some of the greatest flamenco dancers have reached the height of their careers in their sixties! Although you may choose not to perform some of the more vigorous steps, you should still be able to do

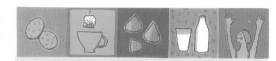

SUPER SHAPER

One of the most effective shaping-up dances is the twist, which first emerged in the 1960s. Some people have suggested that the dance originated as a stylized version of the way rock-and-roll singers swung their hips. It was easy to learn: people were taught to move their feet as if they were trying to stub out a cigarette and move their hips as if they were drying the sweat off their back with a towel—and there was no need for a partner. The twist was, and still is, a great way to lose weight. In the first year of the twist craze, Chubby Checker, who recorded the song "The Twist" in 1960, lost 35 pounds performing the dance to his hit record.

the arm movements and basic footwork as you grow older, and the activity will help you maintain good strength and flexibility.

Flamenco for fitness

Flamenco dance not only is expressive but can also be a great way to get fit and stay in shape. There is a strong emphasis on maintaining an upright position. Women typically hold the back in a slightly arched posture, while men give the impression of height through a straight spine. These effects require both the muscles of the back and the opposing muscle group, the abdominal muscles, to work hard.

A great deal of strength and endurance is required in the leg muscles for the characteristic stamping action (*zapato*). This step demands so much physical force that it was originally performed solely by men, and the women's dance still places a greater emphasis on hand and arm movements. Because the legs include some of the body's largest muscles, they need more oxygen to function. This kind of aerobic training helps to burn excess fat, although a slim or youthful figure is not considered necessary in order to dance the flamenco well.

Many of the women's steps incorporate arm, wrist, and hand movements that reveal the influence of traditional Arabic dance

FLAMENCO AND THE GYPSIES
Andalusian gypsies celebrate festivals with singing and flamenco dancing. The true gypsy flamenco is never choreographed but emerges spontaneously.

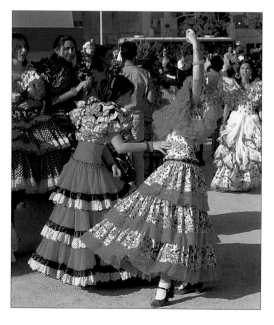

NATIONAL DANCES

Many nationalities around the world celebrate their culture with a form of dance that has been handed down from generation to generation and is often performed at a particular time of year. Many of these dances are linked to traditional folk tales, and some include ancient rituals. For example, in England part of the Morris dancing tradition involves teams of dancers visiting each village in the local area to bring good luck. Other aspects of Morris dancing celebrate fertility. The Maypole dance, for instance, was traditionally an intricate form of courting for young village men and women.

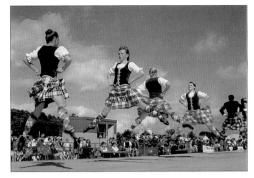

HIGHLAND DANCING
Traditional Scottish dancing from the Highland regions requires a high level of fitness, good flexibility, and very strong inner thigh muscles.

(the Koran forbids a woman to show her legs in public). For example, finger snapping (*pitos*) and rhythmic hand clapping (*palmas*) are important accompaniments to the dance. They help to develop greater flexibility in the wrist and shoulder joints.

BELLY DANCING

Belly dancing originated in the Middle East, but variations can be found all over the world, from North and South America to southern Europe and North Africa. The belly dancing currently popular in the West is considered by many to have originated in Egypt. However, some of the movements were also influenced by Indian, Turkish, and other Middle Eastern forms of dancing.

Traditionally, people in Middle Eastern countries were exposed to dancing and music in every aspect of their lives, regardless of age, fitness, or social class. Dancers of both sexes performed on private occasions—to celebrate a wedding or the birth of a child, for example—as part of religious worship, and sometimes in the streets. Dance was enjoyed instinctively and participated in without inhibitions. Although belly dancing has changed in style over the years, its celebratory qualities remain part of the dance today, and many people from different cultural backgrounds find personal fulfillment in its unrestricted, exuberant, and sensual movements.

Although originally a dance performed by women for other women, nowadays belly dancing can be practiced and enjoyed by

both sexes. It is traditional for men in the Middle East to dance using many belly dancing movements, and men still perform the dance at social functions, including religious festivals. In contrast to the undulating style of the female dance, the men's movements are more athletic.

The notion of maintaining a free spirit and enhancing self-expression is integral to belly dancing and is the primary impulse and energy source of the dance. The distinctive rhythmic patterns of Middle Eastern music provide the atmospheric backdrop for moves that are improvised to create a free interpretation of the music's mood.

Belly dancing for fitness

Belly dancing emphasizes a downward movement of the body, as opposed to the upward lift that characterizes ballet. The feet remain on the ground for most steps, bearing the weight down toward the floor, while the hips and middle section of the body—the main focus of the dance—are vigorously exercised. The dance is expanded and given dynamism by expressive, graceful movements of the arms and hands.

As the middle section of the body strives for maximum movement, the muscles in this region receive a thorough workout. Moving the hips in the characteristic circular action requires hard work. As the hips perform this motion, the middle section of the

continued on page 156

SENSUAL DANCE
Belly dancing is an uninhibited and sensual form of dance that celebrates the body. The dance's sensuality is reflected in the evocative costumes and jewelry worn traditionally as part of the costume.

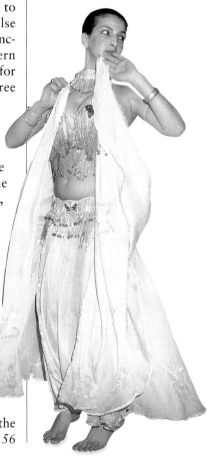

153

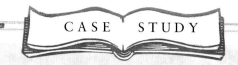

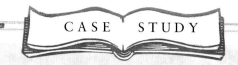

CASE STUDY

An Uninspired Exerciser

Many people begin exercise regimens with the best intentions but find it difficult to maintain interest. Shaping up and staying in shape is a long-term commitment, so it is important to choose an activity about which you are genuinely enthusiastic. Remember that if you are exercising with weight loss in mind, you will have to make changes in your eating habits too.

Rosemary is a 44-year-old senior librarian with three grown children; Jenny, her youngest, has just left home to start college. Until recently Rosemary led quite an active life. She and Jenny, who have a very special relationship, shared much of their free time. Both keen cooks, they used to plan meals together, often experimenting with Thai and Chinese dishes. They also shared a love of evening walks and regularly walked for over an hour at least twice a week. Now that Jenny has moved out, Rosemary has a lot more free time but isn't quite sure what

to do with herself. Her husband, Gerald, has just been promoted and often has to work late. Rosemary has found herself eating alone frequently, and she tends to buy more convenience foods as a result.

Aware that she has slowed down over the past few months and consequently gained some weight, Rosemary has joined an aerobics class at her local gym. However, she has been having difficulty keeping up with the fast pace, and some of the high-impact steps hurt her knees. She also can't help comparing her body with those of other, much younger

women in the class and is feeling less positive about her self-image. She is finding it hard to stay motivated and often decides at the last minute not to attend class, choosing to stay home and watch television instead.

Rosemary has been feeling tired and run down lately and has not been sleeping well. Gerald suggested a visit to the doctor, but she insists that she is not ill enough to bother him. She misses Jenny's vitality and knows that she needs more stimulation in her own life, but increasingly she feels she has no energy to initiate any change at all.

FITNESS
Many people start to slow down as they grow older, and this can lead to weight gain. Keeping active will help to control weight and guard against diseases such as osteoporosis.

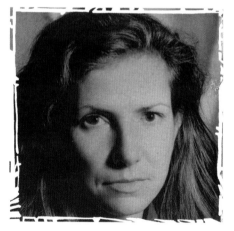

LIFESTYLE
Lack of varied stimulation in daily routine from outside interests and physical pursuits can lead to lethargy, tiredness, frustration, and poor fitness and motivation.

EMOTIONAL HEALTH
Midlife is often a time of change, both in appearance and relationships. This may result in feelings of disorientation, dissatisfaction, and poor self-esteem.

EATING HABITS
Convenience foods are often high in calories and low in essential vitamins. It is healthier to eat a balanced diet with lots of fresh fruits, vegetables, whole grains, and lean protein foods, like fish and chicken breasts.

HEALTH
Some degree of weight gain in middle age is normal but should be kept under control because excess gain is physically unhealthy and contributes to an increased risk of heart disease and other serious illnesses.

154

WHAT SHOULD ROSEMARY DO?

Like many people, Rosemary has not given much thought to the type of exercise she would like to do. To revive her interest and enthusiasm, she needs to find an activity that she genuinely enjoys. There are many forms of exercise that will achieve the same shaping-up results as her aerobics class.

Because Rosemary has always been fascinated with Middle Eastern culture, she recently visited Turkey on vacation and was very taken with the belly dancing she saw there. Classes in belly dancing could be ideal for Rosemary; the pace is less frenetic than that of aerobics, the activity is something new, and it is related to a culture in which she is already interested. Belly dancing will also target the abdominal region, which is one of Rosemary's main problem areas. Not only will she benefit physically from this type of dance, but she will also find an opportunity to step out of her role as mother and wife, allowing her to release mental and physical tension through uninhibited movement.

Rosemary also needs to implement changes in her diet. She should reduce her intake of convenience foods, perhaps cooking interesting and healthful dishes on the weekend and freezing some individual portions to eat during the week whenever her husband works late.

Action Plan

FITNESS

Many forms of dance offer an aerobic workout and muscular toning equal to that gained by more conventional forms of fitness training. Choose an exercise that you enjoy so that you will not be tempted to miss sessions.

EMOTIONAL HEALTH

Find a physical outlet for emotions that is entirely unrelated to your everyday role at work or in the home. Exercise releases "feel good" endorphins and, especially if done in a social environment, can help combat feelings of loneliness.

EATING HABITS

A healthy diet should go hand in hand with increased exercise if a shaping-up program is to succeed. Set aside time for cooking satisfying but low-fat meals. Increase intake of complex carbohydrates to fuel the body for exercise.

HEALTH

Regular exercise reduces the risk of many serious illnesses and can boost energy levels and promote sound sleep. Choose an activity that concentrates on an area you would particularly like to tone and strengthen. Eat more fruits and vegetables to boost the immune system.

LIFESTYLE

Exercise can be a great way to relax and de-stress, as well as tone up physically. By choosing a social exercise such as dancing, you will meet like-minded people and may make some new friends.

HOW THINGS TURNED OUT FOR ROSEMARY

Rosemary joined a belly dancing class, which she found at her local adult education center. Although the class is energetic, she finds it is also therapeutic because it offers a safe environment in which she can express herself without embarrassment. She wants to be able to dance well, which requires good muscle tone. For this reason she has started going to the gym twice a week; after 40 minutes of aerobic work on the running, rowing, and cycling machines, she moves to the weight room to target some of the main muscles used in belly dancing. Because she enjoys the dancing, she doesn't find motivation a problem anymore. Her body is starting to firm up, and she feels much more confident about it.

Rosemary's general feeling of well-being has also increased. She has a lot more energy than before and finds that she now falls asleep easily at night.

Although the exercise classes keep Rosemary busier than she used to be, she has found time to rediscover Asian cooking. Stir-fries, which are quick and easy to prepare, provide her with plenty of fresh vegetables and carbohydrates.

She has persuaded Gerald to get home early at least twice a week. Now he, too, is enjoying the benefits of Rosemary's healthy eating regimen, and he is basking in her positive new outlook.

body has to contract. Consequently, the upper and lower abdominal muscles, the oblique muscles (at the sides of the abdomen), and the muscles in the back all receive a thorough workout. The moves are often repeated, which tones the muscles gradually and enhances their endurance. Repeated exercise of the abdominal muscles, obliques, and back muscles helps to improve the overall tone and shape of this area and also provides an excellent aerobic workout to burn fat from all parts of the body.

The free and unrestricted movement of this oriental dance allows people to let go completely of their external concerns and anxieties. This benefits many aspects of physical health and emotional well-being. It is felt that belly dancing generally helps to raise both self-esteem and confidence.

JAZZ DANCE

Jazz dance provides many of the same physical shaping-up benefits as ballet but with a more contemporary feel and a freer style, which some people find easier to relate to. It originated in the United States and gained widespread popularity in the 1920s during the "Jazz Age." Jazz dance, like the music from which it takes its name, was an Afro-American form developed from a mixture of elements, both African and European. Aspects of ballet and traditional African and Latin American dances have all contributed to its style as well.

ROCK 'N' ROLL
The showing of the film Rock Around the Clock *in the late 1950s was met by a teenage frenzy of enthusiasm for the new dance featured—rock 'n' roll. What started as dancing in the aisles turned into riots in many movie houses in England, making the dance sensation unpopular with adults. The success of rock 'n' roll encouraged music promoters to try to launch other dances; the one shown here is called* The Slug.

Pathway to health
Dance is no longer restricted to special studios; more and more recreation and adult education centers are offering classes in this wonderful exercise at a reasonable cost. It is worth checking with your local center to find out if any forms of dance are taught; many centers allow students to observe a session before committing to a class.

Classes can be a stimulating and sociable way to learn the basics of the dance you are interested in. And the instructor can advise you if the type of dance you have chosen is suitable for your needs, taking into account any existing problems, such as back pain or arthritis.

Jazz dance is very flexible, offering the chance to be funky, smooth, and lyrical; fast and lively; or sophisticated and stylized. The music for it varies in tempo but often includes popular contemporary tracks with lyrics, as opposed to the instrumental music that more often accompanies ballet. The movements in jazz dance are different from those of ballet, although some styles are more influenced than others by balletic choreography and technique. Jazz often incorporates more natural bodily forms, tending to avoid the turned-out and more formally mannered movements of ballet.

A wide range of popular dance styles comes under the jazz dance umbrella, including tap dancing and the jitterbug, so it is certainly possible to find a style to suit your particular interests and needs. The basic requirement is that the dance must be performed to the rhythm of jazz music.

Jazz dance for fitness

Jazz dance can be a highly energetic form of exercise and so is extremely useful for developing stamina. Its links with ballet also mean that it helps develop similarly high levels of flexibility and muscle strength.

Tap dancing provides a particularly good workout for the calves and thighs, while the jitterbug requires a high level of aerobic fitness. Depending on your energy levels, the lifts and swing movements will also demand significant muscle strength.

INDEX

ACKNOWLEDGMENTS

Carroll & Brown Limited
would like to thank
Charteris Sports Centre
Jennie Crewdson
Holmes Place Gym
Iyengar Yoga Institute
  223a Randolph Avenue
  London W9 1NL
Clare and Diego Luzuraga
Gilda Pacitti
Pilates Centre Ltd

Editorial assistance
Denise Alexander
Jennifer Mussett
Laura Price

Photographic assistants
Lee Mcpherson
Colin Tatham

Picture research
Sandra Schneider
Richard Soar

Photograph sources
8 Louvre, Paris, France/Lauros-Giraudon/Bridgeman Art Library, London
9 (top) Galleria dell'Accademia, Venice/Bridgeman Art Library, London
  (bottom) Sporting Pictures (UK) Ltd
19 The Society of Teachers of the Alexander Technique
20 Rolfing Institute
22 ACE Photo Library
23 (top) Popperfoto
  (bottom) REX Features Ltd
25 Mehau Kulyk/Science Photo Library

26 (left) CNRI/Science Photo Library
  (right) Laguna Design/Science Photo Library
27 (top left) Mary Evans Picture Library/Illustrated London News
  (top right) REX Features Ltd
  (bottom) B&C Alexander
28 (top) AKG London/Erich Lessing
  (bottom) Belvoir Castle, Leicestershire/Bridgeman Art Library, London
29 (left) Rodidnice Lobkowicz Coll, Nelahozeves Castle, Czech Republic/Bridgeman Art Library, London
  (middle) Getty Images
  (right) Mary Evans Picture Library
32 (left) REX Features Ltd
  (right) REX Features Ltd
34 (top) AKG London
  (bottom) ACE Photo Agency/Bill Bachmann
42 Images/The Charles Walker Collection
43 (top left) Jules Selmes
  (top right) The Image Bank
  (bottom left) Jules Selmes
45 (left) The Image Bank
  (middle) The Image Bank
  (right) Getty Images
47 The Image Bank
50 Hellerwork, California
53 Scott Camazine/Science Picture Library
63 Sporting Pictures (UK) Ltd
64 Corbis/UPI
69 Art Directors and TRIP/R. Powers
86 Getty Images

87 Manfred Kage/Science Photo Library
91 Images Colour Library
138 ACE Photo Agency/Kevin Phillips
140 Iyengar Yoga Institute
145 James Davis Travel Photography
147 Musee Conde, Chantilly, France/Lauros Giraudon/Bridgeman Art Library, London
148 Getty Images
154 Art Directors and TRIP/T.Bognar
155 Getty Images
155 James Davis Travel Photography
156 Corbis/UPI

Illustrators
Diane Fisher
John Geary
Connie Jude
Bill Piggins
Natasha Stewart
Halli Verinder
Angela Wood

Hair and make-up
Bettina Graham
Kim Menzies

Index
Jennifer Mussett